Steroid Hormones

CROOM HELM BIOLOGY IN MEDICINE SERIES

STEROID HORMONES
D.B. Gower

NEUROTRANSMITTERS AND DRUGS
Zygmunt L. Kruk and Christopher J. Pycock

Steroid Hormones

D. B. Gower

DSc (Lond.) PhD (Lond.), C Chem., FRIC, FI Biol.
Reader in Biochemistry, Guy's Hospital Medical School, London

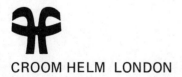

CROOM HELM LONDON

©1979 D.B. Gower
Croom Helm Ltd, 2-10 St John's Road, London SW11

British Library Cataloguing in Publication Data
Gower, D B
   Steroid hormones.
   1. Steroid hormones
   I. Title
   612'.405   QP572.S7

   ISBN 0-85664-838-8
   ISBN 0-85664-855-8 (pbk)

TO DOROTHEA

'that in all things He might have the preeminence'

Colossians 1:18

Printed in Great Britain by
Biddles Ltd, Guildford, Surrey

CONTENTS

PREFACE

This short book on aspects of steroid hormones has stemmed from lectures I give to medical students who take the Basic Medical Sciences course in their first and second years at Guy's Hospital Medical School. The chemical and biochemical aspects are dealt with in the Biochemistry course while the more physiological and endocrinological aspects are pursued in the Human Reproduction and Development course. It was pointed out to me last year that there was no single book in which students could find information on the chemistry, biochemistry, physiology and endocrinology of steroid hormones at the level necessary for the courses they are required to pursue. I welcomed the suggestion that a short book should be written which drew together information from these various disciplines.

It is my experience that some students find the topic of 'steroid hormones' difficult to learn. All too often one hears the cry, 'They all look the same!' Of course this is not surprising, for the compounds are all derived from the same cyclopentanoperhydrophenanthrene nucleus, but it is my hope that, as a result of the way in which the chapters are written and integrated, readers will be able to find a logical sequence in the book and realise the physiological and clinical significance of the steroids.

I am extremely grateful to my wife who has encouraged me throughout the preparation of the work, has typed and retyped the drafts and has helped with the indexing and proof-reading; it is to her that the book is dedicated.

I also express gratitude to Dr H.L.J. Makin of the London Hospital Medical College for making valuable suggestions and criticisms. He is well qualified to do this because he teaches steroid hormone biochemistry during the Basic Medical Sciences course at his own college. Dr G.M. Cooke, a member of my own research group, has kindly given a final, detailed reading to the finished typescript.

Finally, it is a pleasure to acknowledge the help of the Departments of Medical Illustration and Medical Photography of Guy's Hospital for their unfailing help with the illustrations and photographs. Numerous colleagues and publishers have given permission for me to reproduce figures and data from earlier works, and I am grateful to them all. As always, Miss J. Farmer and the staff of the Wills library have provided invaluable help in obtaining books and locating references.

D.B. Gower   April 1979

1 STRUCTURE OF STEROID HORMONES

The parent compound from which all the steroid hormones are ultimately derived is cholesterol. This white, crystalline compound has been known for many centuries and was originally isolated from gall stones; hence the name cholesterol, from *chole*, meaning bile and *stereos*, solid. Cholesterol is a constituent of virtually every animal tissue and occurs partly as the free alcohol and partly esterified with the higher fatty acids.

Figure 1.1: Structural Formulae of Phenanthrene and Cyclopentanoperhydrophenanthrene

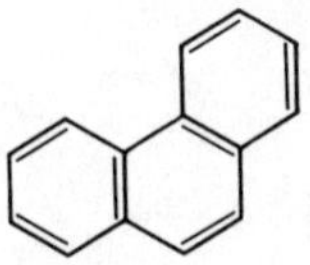

phenanthrene 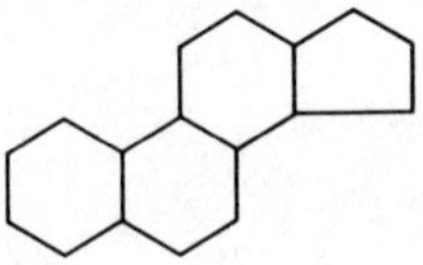   cyclopentanoperhydrophenanthrene

The basic structure to which all the steroids are related is that of fully reduced phenanthrene (perhydrophenanthrene) to which is fused a five-membered ring structure. The complete structure is shown in Figure 1.1 and is known as the cyclopentanoperhydrophenanthrene nucleus. The parent hydrocarbon related to this, and from which cholesterol is derived, is called cholestane. In addition to the fused four-ring structure shown in Figure 1.2, this compound possesses a side-chain eight carbon atoms long, attached at C-17 of ring D. The numbering sequence, also shown in Figure 1.2, is common to all steroids.

Three-dimensional Structure of Steroids

Neither the full formula nor the abbreviated formula (Figure 1.2) for cholestane can adequately represent its structure because it is a three-dimensional molecule, with length approximately 2 nm, width 0.75 nm and thickness 0.45 nm. Figure 1.3 shows that the cyclohexane rings A, B and C are in the 'chair' form, thereby giving rise to corrugations in the structure and thus contributing to the thickness. The alternative 'boat' structure for cyclohexane rings is less stable and does not

11

Figure 1.2: Full and Abbreviated Structures of Cholestane

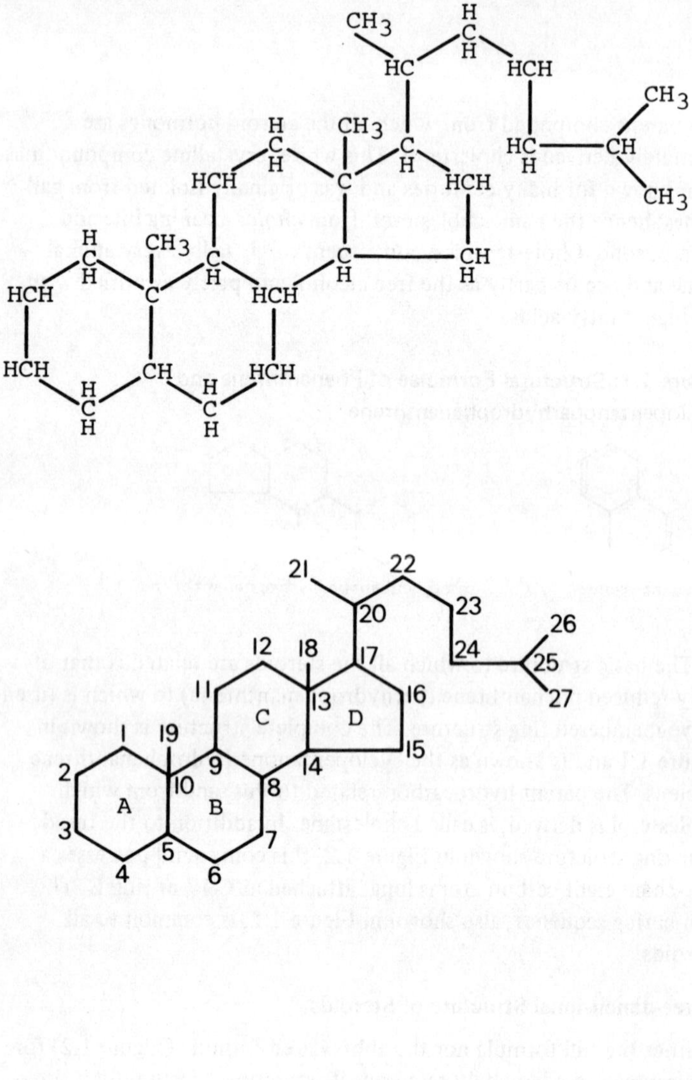

Figure 1.3: Three-dimensional Structures of 5α- and 5β- Cholestane

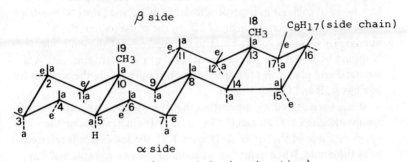

5α- cholestane (trans A:B ring junction)

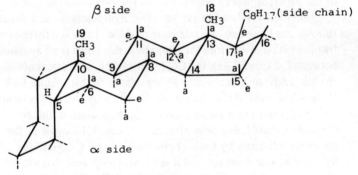

5β- cholestane (cis A:B ring junction)

normally occur. The free valencies of carbon atoms involved in the ring structure are not all in the plane of the molecule (Figure 1.3). One bond of each atom is perpendicular to the plane (axial 'a' bonds), while the other makes an angle of 30° to the plane (equatorial 'e' bonds). This fact also contributes to the thickness of the molecule. It should be noted that, in the special case of the oestrogens, ring A is aromatic and planar and this unsaturation results also in the coplanarity of rings A, B and C.

It has been agreed by convention that the so-called 'angular' methyl groups attached at C-10 and C-13 and the side-chain all define the upper or β side of the molecule (Figure 1.3); the lower side is referred to as the α side. When depicting a steroid in the two-dimensional way, it is conventional to show β groups, which lie above the plane of the paper, as full lines (———) and to show α groups, lying below the plane of the paper, as broken lines (– – – –).

Cholestane is related to various other hydrocarbons, and virtually all steroids can be defined by reference to these. Thus, if a three-carbon fragment is removed from the cholestane side-chain (i.e., by fission between C-24 and C-25), the C_{24} hydrocarbon, cholane, is obtained; the bile acids, such as cholic acid, are related to this (Figure 1.4). Removal of most of the cholestane side-chain by cleavage between C-20 and C-22, results in pregnane, the C_{21} hydrocarbon; to this compound, the corticosteroids and progesterone are related. Removal of the complete side-chain by fission between C-17 and C-20 leads to the C_{19} hydrocarbon, androstane, and it is to this compound that the androgens, such as testosterone, are related. Finally, removal of the methyl group at C-10 of androstane gives rise to oestrane, to which the oestrogens are related. Figure 1.4 illustrates these structural relationships and shows one example of a biologically important steroid in each case. It should be noted that the systematic name of steroids refers to the parent hydrocarbon. For example, cholesterol is 5-cholesten-3β-ol, the 'en' in the stem name indicating that unsaturation, $-CH=CH-$, is present in the molecule, while the number outside the stem indicates the position of unsaturation – in this case at C-5 and C-6. By convention, only the lower number is required, which in this text will be shown outside the stem, following the rules of the International Union of Pure and Applied Chemistry (IUPAC). In cases of ambiguity, as for example in oestradiol-17β, the double bond between C-5 and C-10 is indicated 5(10). The use of Δ to indicate unsaturation, e.g., Δ^4, is now not permitted in systematic nomenclature. Where more than one double bond is present, these are indicated in (say) oestradiol-17β as

Figure 1.4:

Structural Relationships between Cholestane (C_{27}), Cholane (C_{24}), Pregnane (C_{21}), Androstane (C_{19}) and Oestrane (C_{18}). Examples of biologically important steroids related to each parent hydrocarbon are also shown

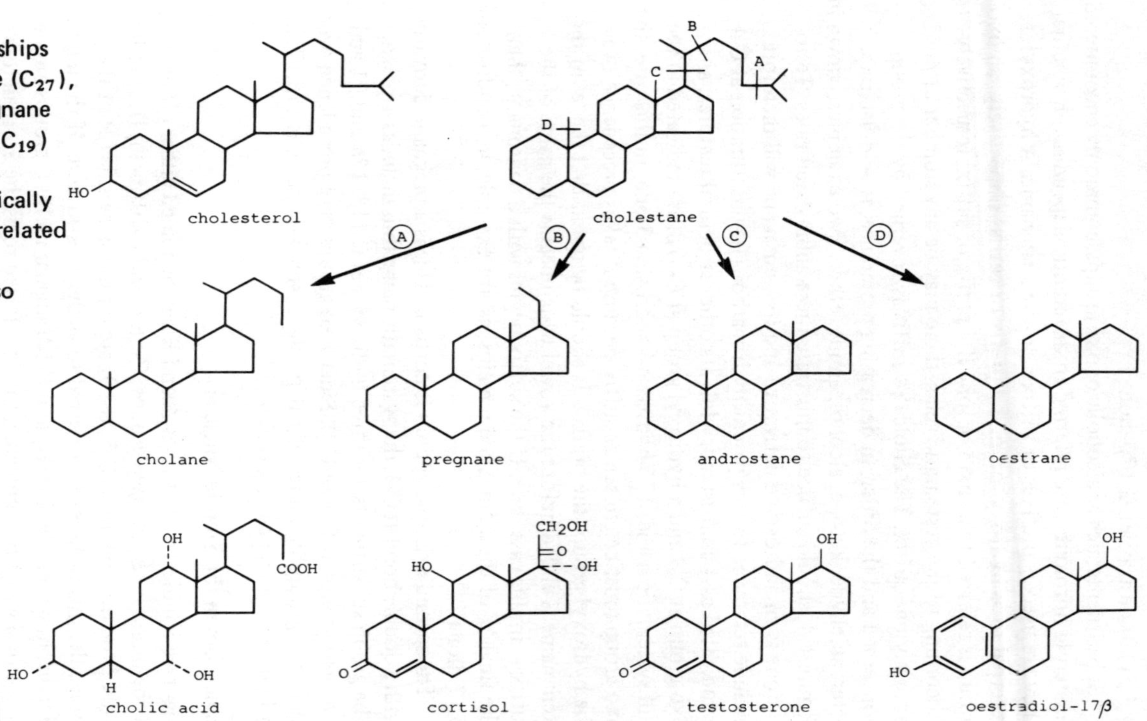

cholesterol

(A) (B) cholestane (C) (D)

cholane

pregnane

androstane

oestane

cholic acid

cortisol

testosterone

oestradiol-17β

1,3,5(10)-oestratrien-3,17β-diol.

Substituents such as alcoholic or oxo groups, commonly encountered in steroid hormones, are referred to differently depending on whether they are used as prefixes or suffixes to the stem name. A hydroxyl is referred to as hydroxy- or -ol if a prefix or suffix, respectively; an oxo group is referred to as oxo- or -one if a prefix or suffix, respectively. According to the systematic rules, there may be any number of prefixes but only one suffix. The choice of suffix is governed by the group concerned and the order, in decreasing preference, is acid, lactone, ester, aldehyde, ketone, alcohol, amine, ether. Two examples, shown in Figure 1.4, should suffice to illustrate these abbreviated rules. Testosterone is an androstane derivative and its stem name will therefore include reference to this parent hydrocarbon. Its unsaturation at C-4 is indicated as 4-androstene, while its other structural features, an oxo group at C-3 and a hydroxyl group at C-17β, are indicated in the full systematic name, 17β-hydroxy-4-androsten-3-one. In this case, the oxo group must be chosen as suffix because it takes precedence over the hydroxyl group (the prefix). It should be noted that the 'e' of the stem name is elided before the vowel which begins the name of the suffix — in this case -one. If the suffix begins with a consonant, then the final 'e' of the stem name remains, as, for example, in 4-androstene-3,17-dione.

The second example chosen is cortisol. This is a pregnane derivative with a double bond at C-4; the systematic name thus includes 4-pregnene. The group substituents are three hydroxyls at C-11β, 17α and 21 and two oxo groups at C-3 and 20. Since oxo groups take precedence over hydroxyl groups in choice of suffix, the systematic name is 11β,17α,21-trihydroxy-4-pregnene-3,20-dione.

Isomerism in the Steroid Nucleus

Figure 1.3 indicates that rings A and B can be joined either *cis* or *trans*. If the union is *cis*, the two groups, C-5(H) and C-10(methyl), at either end of the ring junction (C-5, C-10) are on the same side (β) of the molecule; this is therefore referred to as the 5β-structure. If the union is *trans*, however, the C-5(H) and C-10(angular methyl) groups are on opposite sides of the molecule; this is referred to as the 5α-structure. Obviously, no isomerism occurs at C-5 if there is unsaturation in that position or, as indicated above, if ring A is aromatic. This type of isomerism means that the various parent hydrocarbons — cholestane, pregnane, etc. — can exist in both the 5α- and 5β-forms. It also means that reduction of a compound which has unsaturation at C-4 (e.g., 4-

Figure 1.5: The Reduction of 5α-androstane-3,17-dione, Illustrating Isomerism at C-3

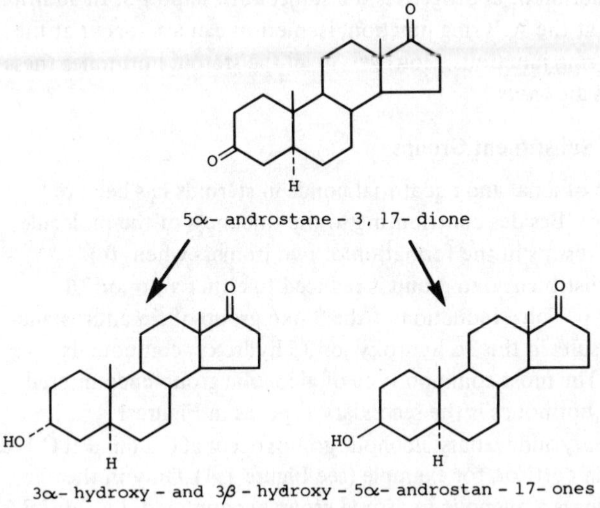
O
O
H
5α- androstane - 3, 17- dione
O
HO
H
O
HO
H
3α- hydroxy - and 3β - hydroxy - 5α- androstan - 17- ones

Figure 1.6: The Reduction of Progesterone, Illustrating Isomerism at C-20

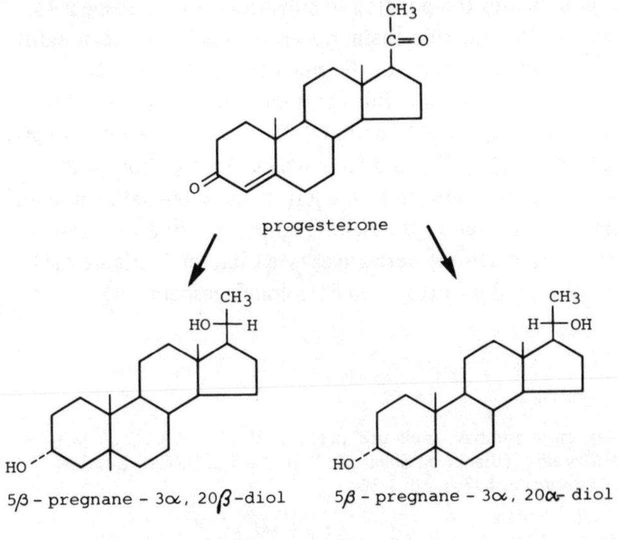
CH3
C=O
O
progesterone
CH3
HO H
HO
CH3
H OH
HO
5β - pregnane - 3α, 20β-diol
5β - pregnane - 3α, 20α- diol

androstenedione) will give rise to two isomers – in this case, 5α-andro-stane-3,17-dione and 5β-androstane-3,17-dione (see Figure 5.3). Enzymic reduction of androgens is the subject of Chapter 5. In addition to isomerism at the A:B ring junction, isomerism can also occur at the B:C and C:D ring junctions. However, in all the steroid hormones these ring junctions are *trans*.

Isomerism of Substituent Groups

The existence of axial and equatorial bonds in steroids has been re-ferred to above. Besides contributing to the thickness of the molecule, this property results in the formation of two isomers when, for example, a substituent oxo group is reduced to either a 3α- or 3β-alcoholic group. Thus, reduction of the 3-oxo group of 5α-androstane-3,17-dione results in the 3α-hydroxy- or 3β-hydroxy- compounds (Figure 1.5). The most common type of alcoholic group encountered in the steroid hormones is the secondary type, as in Figure 1.4, although primary and tertiary alcoholic groups occur at C-21 and at C-17α, respectively, in cortisol, for example (see Figure 1.4). Only in the oestrogen series is a phenolic hydroxyl group encountered, i.e., at C-3 of the aromatic A ring (see Figure 1.4).

Isomerism in the Side-chain at C-17

A detailed discussion of this topic is outside the scope of the present text but is dealt with elsewhere (see Kellie, 1975). As seen earlier, the use of α- and β- indicates the position of substituents with respect to the steroid nucleus; for the side-chain, however, this is not meaningful because the asymmetric C-atoms of the side-chain may not them-selves lie in the plane of the ring. But for isomerism at C-20, it is still accepted practice to employ 20α- and 20β-. Thus, progesterone can give rise to 5β-pregnane-3α,20α-diol and 5β-pregnane-3α,20β-diol. In the 20α-isomer the H atom is written to the left of the side-chain while, in the 20β-isomer, it is written to the right (Figure 1.6). In a similar way, reduced cortisol and cortisone derivatives (see Chapter 5, Figure 5.1) are referred to as α- and β- cortols and cortolones, respectively.

Reference

Kellie, A.E., 'Structure and Nomenclature' in H.L.J. Makin (ed.), *Biochemistry of Steroid Hormones* (Blackwell Scientific Publications, Oxford-London-Edinburgh-Melbourne, 1975), pp. 1-16.

2 PHYSIOLOGICAL ACTIONS: CORRELATION OF STRUCTURE AND FUNCTION

The Corticosteroids

The group of steroids called the corticosteroids are formed in the adrenal cortex and are usually classified under two headings — (a) the 17-hydroxylated corticosteroids and (b) the 17-deoxycorticosteroids — depending on the presence or absence of a 17α-hydroxyl group. Although there is some overlap of function between the two groups (as will be seen later), the 17-hydroxylated compounds are gluco-corticoids, while the 17-deoxy compounds are mineralocorticoids.

The Glucocorticoids

Figure 2.1 gives the structures of naturally-occurring steroids in this group, such as cortisol, and also some synthetic compounds, such as prednisolone. They exert powerful effects on a wide variety of meta-bolic events. Overall effects on carbohydrate and nitrogen metabolism result in an increase in glucose production; thus the actions of the glucocorticoids are antagonistic to those of insulin. This is accom-plished by the induction of many of the glycolytic enzymes and aminotransferases (gluconeogenic mechanisms).

Figure 2.2 illustrates, in abbreviated form, the metabolism of glucose to pyruvate (the glycolysis pathway) and the complete oxidation of the latter via the reactions of the tricarboxylic acid (TCA) cycle. Transamination of alanine results in the formation of pyruvate, while aspartate and glutamate can be converted into oxaloacetate and 2-oxoglutarate, respectively (both TCA cycle intermediates), by means of the appropriate aminotransferases. Through the action of the enzyme phosphoenol pyruvate carboxykinase, in association with guanidine triphosphate, oxaloacetate can be converted to phosphoenol pyruvate (PEP), thus by-passing the irreversible step in the glycolytic sequence, PEP → pyruvate. The 11-oxygenated corticosteroids, such as cortisol, are known to bring about the induction of several amino-transferases in the liver (see Figure 2.2) and also many other enzymes, including PEP carboxykinase, pyruvate carboxylase, fructose-1,6-diphosphatase and glucose-6-phosphatase. The overall result is the synthesis of glucose from amino acids.

There are two more liver enzymes involved in the metabolism of

Figure 2.1: Structural Formulae of Naturally-occurring Corticosteroids. The synthetic steroids, prednisolone and dexamethasone, are also represented

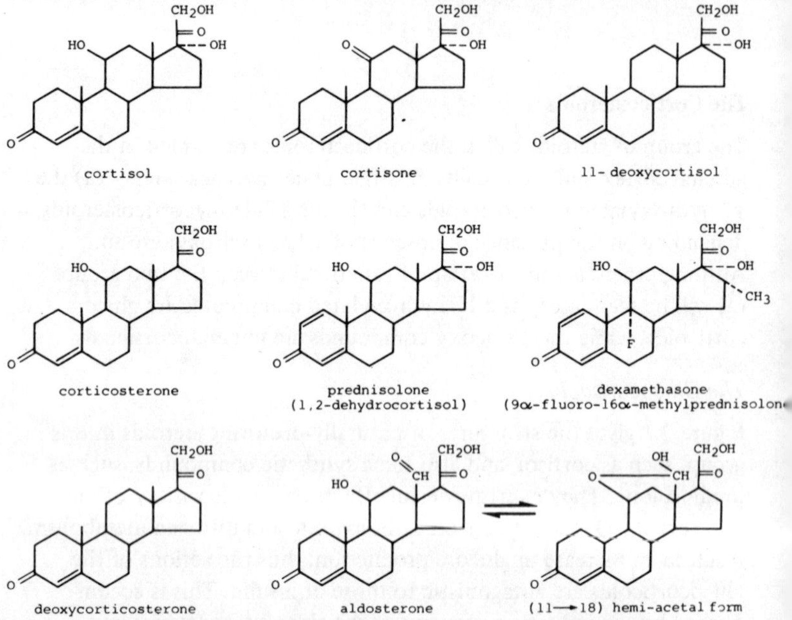

cortisol

cortisone

11- deoxycortisol

corticosterone

prednisolone
(1,2-dehydrocortisol)

dexamethasone
(9α-fluoro-16α-methylprednisolone)

deoxycorticosterone

aldosterone

(11→18) hemi-acetal form

specific amino acids, which are induced by glucocorticoids. These are tyrosine aminotransferase (TAT) and tryptophan pyrrolase (TP), and measurements of their activity in liver preparations are utilised extensively in determining the potency of steroids with possible glucocorticoid action. TAT catalyses the transamination of tyrosine in the presence of the oxo-acid acceptor, 2-oxoglutarate (Figure 2.3), and results in the formation of p-hydroxyphenyl pyruvate. This is further oxidised to homogentisate, which is converted ultimately to fumarate and acetoacetate. This means that tyrosine is both a glucogenic and an oxogenic amino acid. The time of induction of TAT is between five and twelve hours. TP, which is induced in three to five hours, is concerned with the initial oxidation of tryptophan to N-formylkynurenine (Figure 2.3). Further reactions result ultimately in the formation of acetoacetate; thus, tryptophan is an oxogenic amino acid.

In addition to the stimulation of hepatic gluconeogenesis, other effects, such as increased urea and ketone body synthesis, also occur as a consequence of increased mobilisation to the liver of amino acids and free fatty acids, respectively. It is therefore appropriate that the

Figure 2.2: Abbreviated Scheme Showing the Influence ⊕ of Glucocorticoids on Gluconeogenic Enzymes

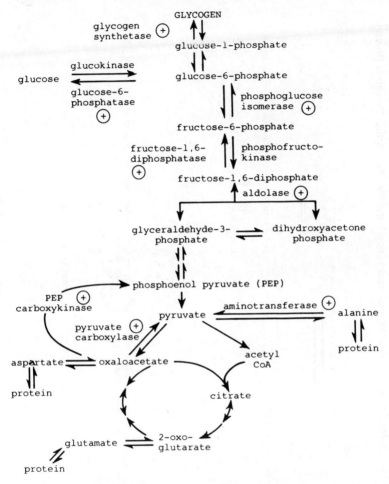

urea cycle enzymes, arginine synthetase, argininosuccinate lyase and arginase, are all induced in two to four days to cope with the ammonia resulting from the deamination of the amino acids. The induction times of the glycolytic enzymes are in the range three to six days except for 3-phosphoglyceraldehyde dehydrogenase and pyruvate carboxylase, which are affected in as short a time as four to eight hours.

The diversity of metabolic effects of glucocorticoids is further exemplified by the fact that, in adipose tissue, muscle and lymphatic

Figure 2.3: Reactions Catalysed by L-tyrosine Aminotransferase (upper) and by Tryptophan Pyrrolase (lower)

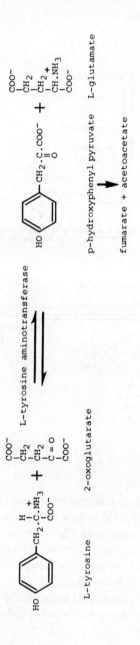

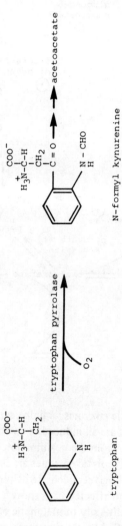

tissue, glucose utilisation is reduced. The increase in free fatty acid release from adipose tissue results in increased ketone body synthesis in the liver, as mentioned earlier.

Glucocorticoids and the Inflammatory Response. Another important effect of glucocorticoids is their suppression of the inflammatory reaction which occurs in response to tissue injury. Fibroblasts are known to be important target tissues of cortisol and synthetic glucocorticoids such as prednisolone (Figure 2.1) and these steroids can cause morphological changes in fibroblasts *in vivo*. Thus, they inhibit wound healing both through suppression of proliferation and the inflammatory response (which are characteristic of the first stage of healing) and through inhibition of the synthesis of collagen and mucopolysaccharides (which are necessary for the second stage of healing).

The inflammatory reaction also occurs as a response to more general allergic conditions like hay-fever, asthma and rheumatoid arthritis. While the mechanism of the beneficial effects of glucocorticoids in such conditions is poorly understood, it seems that their ability to suppress the liberation of histamine and serotonin is important. Thus, the vasodilatory and permeability effects of the two amines on the capillary blood system are reduced.

The Mineralocorticoids

In contrast to the diversity of actions of the glucocorticoids, the actions of the mineralocorticoids, such as aldosterone and deoxycorticosterone (DOC), are confined to effects on salt and water metabolism. In response to a lowered plasma sodium-ion concentration, the formation of angiotensin II (see Chapter 6) is stimulated, and this, in turn, results in increased secretion of aldosterone by the zona glomerulosa cells of the adrenal cortex, whereupon sodium-ions are retained by the renal tubules. Chloride and bicarbonate ions are also increasingly reabsorbed by the cells of the renal distal tubules, sweat glands, salivary glands and intestinal mucosa. An increase in plasma and intracellular potassium-ion concentration, however, is known to decrease aldosterone secretion by the adrenals and results in raised excretion of potassium-ion in the urine.

Correlation of the Structure of Corticosteroids and Their Physiological Actions

The basic structural requirement for a compound to possess corticosteroid activity is that it should be a C_{21} compound with a $-CO \cdot CH_2OH$

Table 2.1: Relative Biological Potencies of Corticosteroids, in Relation to Structure

Corticosteroid	17-OH	21-OH	11-OH	Glycogen deposition[a]	Anti-inflammatory effect[a]	Salt-retaining effect[a]
Cortisol	+	+	+	1.0	1.0	1.0
Cortisone[b]	+	+	+	0.65	0.013	0.66
Corticosterone	−	+	+	0.3	0.03	1.6
Prednisolone	+	+	+	4	3	1
Dexamethasone	+	+	+	17	28	0.1
Aldosterone	−	+	(+)[c]	0.3	0	300
Deoxycorticosterone	−	+	−	0	0	10

a The amount of liver glycogen deposited 60 min after steroid injections to adrenalectomised rats was compared with that obtained after administering 100 μg cortisol/100 g. Anti-inflammatory activity was estimated by the 'granuloma pouch test', which measures the effect of different steroids on the weight of a granuloma (a fibrous deposit) induced by an implanted irritant. Salt-retaining effect of steroids was evaluated from the amounts of sodium- and potassium-ions appearing in the urine of adrenalectomised rats on controlled salt and water allowance.

b The biological effects of cortisone, which has an oxo group at C-11, are due to partial conversion to cortisol (11-hydroxyl group) by 11β-hydroxysteroid dehydrogenase activity.

c Aldosterone normally occurs in the hemi-acetal form and does not possess an 11β-hydroxyl group.

Source: Quantitative data taken from D. Schulster, S. Burstein and B.A. Cooke, Molecular Endocrinology of the Steroid Hormones (1976), by permission of the authors and John Wiley & Sons, London-New York-Sydney-Toronto.

side-chain attached at C-17. Reduction at C-20 causes marked loss in activity and is one of the ways by which deactivation takes place *in vivo* (see Chapter 5). In addition, there must be a 4-en-3-oxo configuration in ring A (Figure 2.1). Glucocorticoid activity requires an oxygen function at C-11 as, for example, in cortisol, which has an 11β-hydroxyl group. Cortisone, although having an 11-oxo group, has some biological activity *in vivo* (Table 2.1) because of the presence of the enzyme 11β-hydroxysteroid dehydrogenase. The presence of a hydroxyl group at C-17 enhances glucocorticoid activity but, in contrast, hydroxyl groups at C-11 and C-17 decrease mineralocorticoid activity, while a 21-hydroxyl group is necessary as, for example, in DOC and aldosterone (Figure 2.1).

The most potent mineralocorticoid, aldosterone, is a special case because it possesses characteristic structural features of both a glucocorticoid (11β-hydroxyl) and a mineralocorticoid (21-hydroxyl). However, in the natural state, aldosterone occurs as the hemi-acetal form, as a result of the close spatial proximity of the 11β-hydroxyl and 18-aldehyde group (Figure 2.1). This interaction results in a masking of glucocorticoid activity (normally anticipated for an 11β-hydroxyl group), while still allowing the mineralocorticoid effect of the 21-hydroxyl group. It is clear that in aldosterone the presence of the 18-aldehyde group confers about 90 per cent of the mineralocorticoid effect. The data in Table 2.1 illustrate the physiological effects of the corticosteroids.

The Androgens

The androgens comprise a group of C_{19} steroids which are secreted to a large extent by the Leydig cells of the interstitial tissue of the testes and to a lesser extent by the adrenals and ovaries. There is some evidence that the Sertoli cells of the seminiferous tubules can also synthesise and secrete testosterone.

Androgens exert numerous diverse effects. *In utero*, irrespective of genetic sex, development of male reproductive organs occurs if the foetus produces androgens. Normally, this only occurs in genetic males and it is at puberty when androgen masculinising effects are manifested most markedly. They are involved with the normal functioning and structure of the prostate gland and seminal vesicles — in particular, with spermatogenesis and with citric acid and fructose formation. Further, at puberty there is an increase in the size of the testes, scrotum, penis, seminal vesicles, prostate, vas deferens and epididymis.

The anabolic effects of androgens are also noted at this time in that there is an increase in muscle protein, reflected in an increased urinary creatinine, a decrease in urinary nitrogen excretion without an increase in blood urea. These effects, including those on bone, give rise to the dramatic increases in height and weight noted in boys at puberty.

Effects of androgens on non-sexual organs include those on the length of the vocal chords, resulting in deepening of the voice, and on the kidneys. These are larger in men than in women and numerous enzymes are increased in quantity, viz., acid phosphatase, β-glucuronidase and those involved in nitrogen metabolism, amino acid oxidase and arginase. A further well-known effect is noted at puberty — the increase in sebum production as a result of increased activity of the sebaceous glands occasionally leading to the troublesome problem of acne. Sexual, axillary and facial hair-growth is also androgen-dependent.

Correlation of Steroid Structure and Androgenic Potency

Assessment of the androgenicity of compounds is commonly carried out using castrated rats or mice, allowing time for the effects of the previously circulating androgens to wear off and then studying the increase in weight of prostate and seminal vesicles after administration of graded doses of test compound. Using these and other assays, it has been possible to obtain a reasonably clear definition of the structure for a steroid if it is to possess androgenic activity.

The major naturally-occurring androgens are testosterone, 5α-dihydrotestosterone (5α-DHT) and 5α-androstane-$3\alpha,17\beta$-diol, with 4-androstenedione and dehydroepiandrosterone (DHA) having only weak activity (Figure 2.4). It must be remembered, however, that androgens occur in plasma in very variable concentrations and that, in some circumstances (i.e., DHA-producing adrenal tumours), the most potent androgens are not always the most physiologically important.

A study of the structures of these compounds reveals a number of structural characteristics:

(1)   They are all C_{19} steroids.
(2)   The presence of a 17β-hydroxyl group is a requirement because, if this is oxidised to a 17-oxo group (as in 4-androstenedione), there is a loss of approximately 80 per cent in androgenic potency. Alternatively, if a 17α-hydroxyl group is present (as in epitestosterone) or if the steroid is devoid of an oxygen function at C-17 (as in 4,16-androstadien-3-one), then the steroids concerned have little or no androgenicity.

Figure 2.4: Structural Formulae of some C$_{19}$ Steroids

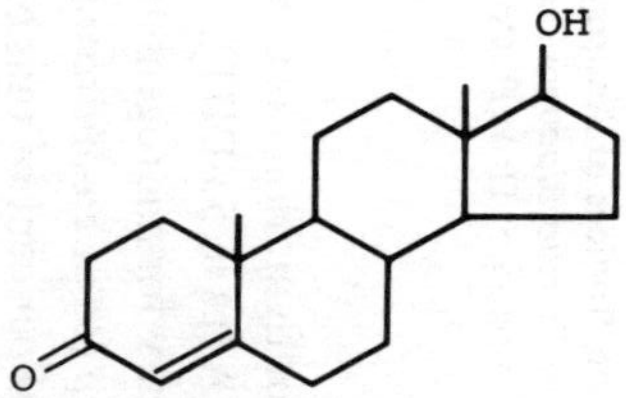

testosterone

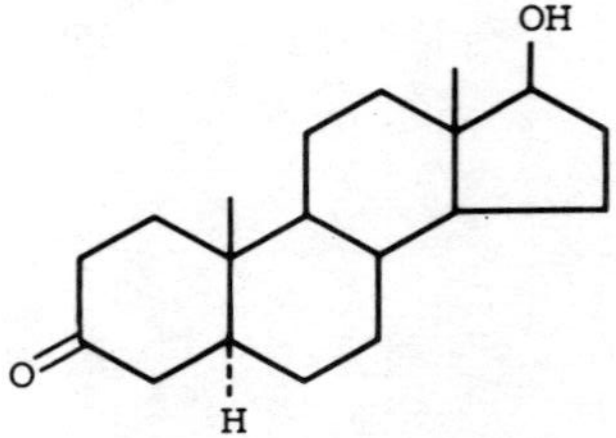

5α – dihydrotestosterone

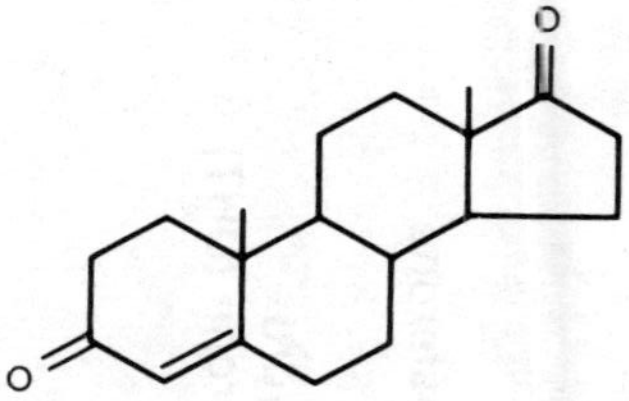

4 – androstenedione

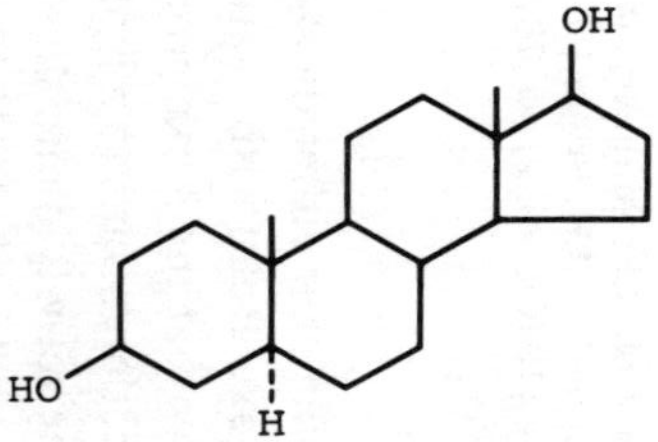

5α– androstane–3β, 17β–diol

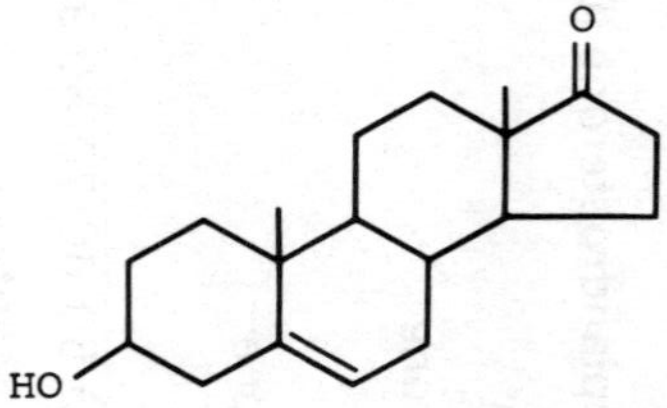

dehydroepiandrosterone

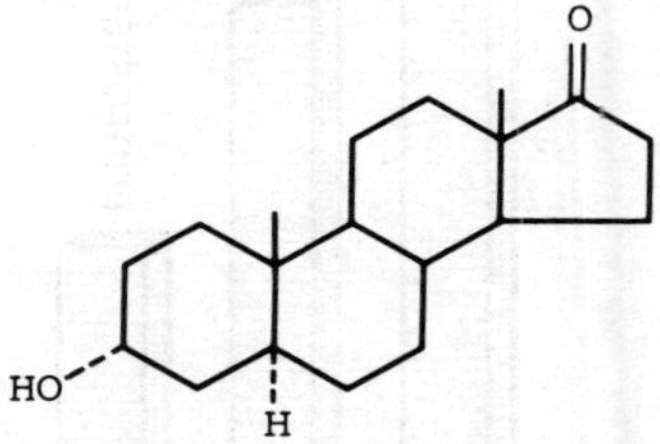

androsterone

Figure 2.5: Androgenic Potency Relative to Testosterone (≡ 100 per cent) of Some C_{19} Steroids

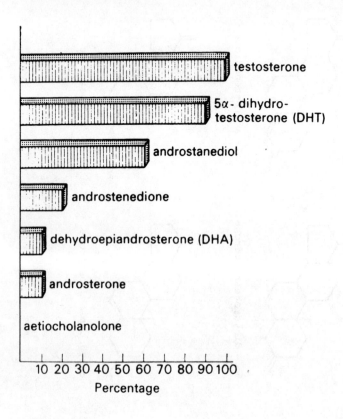

Source: Reprinted from I.F. Sommerville & W.P. Collins, 'Indices of Androgen Production in Women' in M.H. Briggs (ed.), *Advances in Steroid Biochemistry and Pharmacology* (1970), vol. 2, pp. 267-314, by permission of Dr W.P. Collins and Academic Press.

(3)   They should have either the 4-en-3-oxo configuration (as in testosterone) or a 3-oxo group with a saturated ring A (as in 5α-DHT). Figure 2.5 shows that the 3-oxo group is necessary for androgenicity because, if reduction occurs to a hydroxyl group (as in 5α-androstane-3α,17β-diol), the activity diminishes to about 60 per cent of that of testosterone, even though the 17β-hydroxyl group is still intact. Further, a compound with a 5-ene-3β-hydroxy configuration, such as

DHA, has limited potency.

(4)   If ring A is saturated, then it is the 5α-isomer which is found to possess slightly higher androgenicity (although this is very small) than the corresponding 5β-isomer; compare the structures of androsterone (3α,5α-) and aetiocholanolone (3α,5β-).

It should be noted that the androgenicities of different compounds vary to some extent depending on the method of assay. This is particularly important in the case of 5α-DHT where, in some assays, it has been shown to be a more potent androgen than testosterone. Indeed, it is now generally considered that 5α-DHT is the active form of testosterone in some target organs (see Chapter 4).

The Oestrogens

The oestrogens are concerned with the normal growth and development of the female reproductive tract. Together with the C_{21} steroid, progesterone, they control the oestrous and menstrual cycles, and inhibit gonadotrophin production by the anterior pituitary. During pregnancy, gestation is maintained by oestrogens and progesterone working synergistically. These topics are described in more detail in Chapters 6 and 7.

Oestrogens also have extragenital effects; at puberty, they are responsible for breast development and for the typical female body shape. Effects on calcium and nitrogen metabolism are also noticed in that calcification of epiphyseal cartilage is stimulated and nitrogen is retained through mild anabolic effects. After the menopause, women often go into negative calcium balance and signs of osteoporosis are evident, as a result of the decline in plasma oestrogen levels which no longer antagonise the osteoporotic effects of corticosteroids. The bones become more fragile and this leads to the distinct possibility of fractures. Undoubtedly, this is due to parathormone inducing calcium resorption from bone, effects which are normally controlled in younger women by oestrogen.

The effects of oestrogens on oral structures have been studied for many years, and it is known that they influence the growth of the oral epithelium. Some experiments have indicated that oestriol increases the activity of cells in the buccal epithelium; although the increases were much smaller than those in the vagina, the results show that the oral epithelium is a target tissue for oestrogens. Similarly, in other work, injected [³H] oestradiol-17β was shown to bind to oral tissues such as buccal mucosa and gingiva.

Figure 2.6: Structural Formulae of Oestrogens

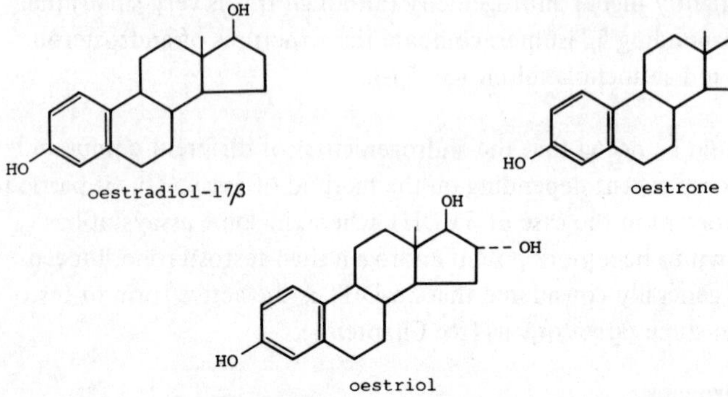

oestradiol-17β

oestrone

oestriol

Figure 2.6 shows the structures of the important oestrogens. Oestradiol-17β is the most potent of the group, but oxidation to oestrone or further hydroxylation at C-16 to give oestriol reduce oestrogenicity. The activity of other hydroxylated, oxygenated or methylated oestrogens is fairly small, and these compounds are mainly regarded as catabolic products (see Chapter 5).

3 BIOSYNTHESIS OF CORTICOSTEROIDS, ANDROGENS AND OESTROGENS

In early experiments which were designed to investigate the biosynthesis of steroid hormones, steroids were either incubated with preparations of steroid-transforming tissues, such as adrenal cortex, or administered *in vivo* to human subjects or animals. In such experiments it was difficult to distinguish the metabolites of the administered steroid from those present endogenously, i.e., before the experiment had begun. In an attempt to obviate this difficulty, large amounts of substrates were used, leading to the second difficulty that such large quantities might cause disturbance of the normal steroid metabolism. More physiological experiments had to await the synthesis of steroids which were isotopically labelled with ^{14}C or ^3H, and it was after this that numerous studies were performed to unravel the complexities of the biosynthesis of steroid hormones. More recently, isotopically labelled steroids of extremely high specific activity (i.e., of the order of 150 Ci/mmol) have become available, and this has meant that it is possible to administer only picogramme quantities of labelled steroid to the subject or animal concerned, without any physiological disturbance.

Detailed discussion of the methods available for studying steroid metabolism is beyond the scope of this book and only a brief indica- ation will be given here. The subject is dealt with in detail, however, by Gower (1975), Gower & Fotherby (1975) and Schulster, Burstein & Cooke (1976). For *in vivo* studies, the labelled steroid is either injected or infused into a vein over a given period. Thereafter, blood is withdrawn at suitable intervals and analysed for the labelled steroid and its metabolites. It is also usual to collect samples of urine from the experimental subject because steroid metabolites, often conjugated as sulphates or glucuronides, are excreted via the kidneys (see Chapter 5). However, if information about a particular organ is required, the labelled steroid is usually infused into the arterial blood supply and the venous blood subsequently analysed for labelled metabolites.

Experiments *in vitro* are performed using homogenates or sub- cellular fractions (mitochondria, microsomes, cytosol) of steroid- transforming tissues such as adrenal cortex, testes, liver, etc. The tissue preparation is then incubated under suitable conditions with the isotopically labelled steroid substrate for either fixed or varied times. In earlier experiments, incubation times of up to eight hours have been used but, in more recent work, periods of up to 60 minutes are commonly employed. For studies of the conversion of cholesterol into pregnenolone, incubation times of only a few seconds are required because the intermediates turn over so rapidly.

In such isolated tissue preparations, it is necessary to supplement the incubation medium with required cofactors. Steroid metabolites tend to build up in static incubations, and it is argued by some that steroid biosynthetic pathways could thus be altered artificially. As an alternative, and possibly more physiological method, the technique of 'superfusion' was devised. This consists of a small glass tube with a sintered filter at one end, on which thin slices of tissue are placed. A suitable buffered medium containing isotopically labelled steroid is then pumped over the tissue at a constant rate and the effluent liquid analysed. Such a system more closely approximates the physiological situation where the steroid metabolites are continually being removed from an organ in the venous blood. The technique of superfusion is being effectively used in the study of the control of steroid biosynthesis by corticotrophin, gonadotrophins and prostaglandins, which can be included in the 'superfusing' medium.

Biosynthesis of the Steroid Hormones

Evidence obtained both *in vivo* and *in vitro* has clearly shown that cholesterol is the parent compound from which the corticosteroids, androgens and oestrogens are formed biosynthetically. The pathway of formation of cholesterol from acetate is also well known but will not be discussed here because it is dealt with adequately in books of general biochemistry. It appears that the cholesterol pool gives rise directly to the steroid hormones, but is rapidly replenished by conversion of acetate. The series of reactions involved is summarised in Figure 3.1 and will be discussed in some detail. In summary, most of the side-chain of the C_{27} steroid, cholesterol, is removed to form the C_{21} steroid, pregnenolone. This then gives rise to the corticosteroids in the adrenal cortex and to the C_{19} steroids, the androgens, when the remaining side-chain is removed. Further transformations including the removal of the angular methyl group from C-10, result in the C_{18} steroids, the oestrogens.

Conversion of Cholesterol to Pregnenolone. It is generally accepted that the trophic hormones act between cholesterol and pregnenolone,

Figure 3.1: Summary of Steroid-hormone Biosynthesis from Cholesterol

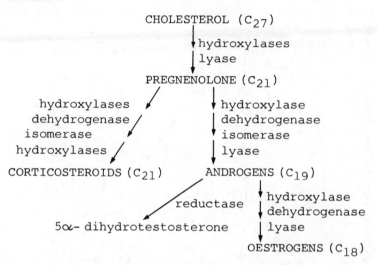

thereby influencing the biosynthesis of most of the steroid hormones. Furthermore, one of the steps is rate-limiting and it is probably for these two reasons that this series of steps has been, and is still being, actively investigated.

The conversion of cholesterol to pregnenolone occurs in the mitochondria of all steroid hormone-producing tissues. Although numerous mechanisms have been proposed, it is currently thought that cholesterol is hydroxylated first at C-22 (Figure 3.2), then further at C-20, and that cleavage of the side-chain fragment occurs between C-20 and C-22 by means of the C-20,22 lyase. At the time of writing it is thought probable that a concerted series of reactions takes place while the substrate and intermediates are bound to the enzyme surface. This occurs as a complex of two hydroxylases and the lyase bound to the inner mitochondrial membrane and requires cytochrome P-450, NADPH and O_2 for activity; the complex is thus of the 'mixed function' oxygenase type. The side-chain fragment produced is isocaproic aldehyde (4-methylpentanal) but this is rapidly oxidised to isocaproic acid (4-methylpentanoic acid) in many tissues.

Correlation of Structure and Function of the Adrenals. The adrenal cortex consists of three histologically defined zones (Figure 3.3) —

Figure 3.2: The Probable Sequence of Reactions Involved in the Conversion of Cholesterol into Pregnenolone

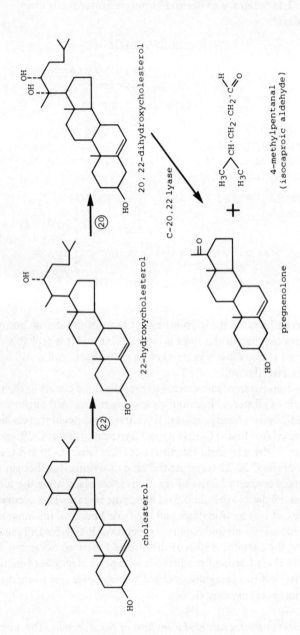

cholesterol

22-hydroxycholesterol

20, 22-dihydroxycholesterol

C-20, 22 lyase

pregnenolone

4-methylpentanal
(isocaproic aldehyde)

Figure 3.3: Histology of the Adrenal Cortex and the Effect of ACTH

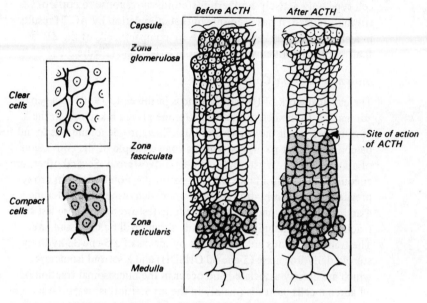

Source: Reprinted from D.B. Gower, 'Control of Steroidogenesis', in H.L.J. Makin (ed.), *Biochemistry of the Steroid Hormones* (1975), pp. 127-47, by permission of Blackwell Scientific Publications, Oxford-London-Edinburgh-Melbourne.

the zona glomerulosa (ZG), the zona fasciculata (ZF) and the zona reticularis (ZR). In man, the ZG consists not so much of a discrete band of tissue but of pockets or islands of cells, so that in many places the ZF extends to the capsule. It is the cells of the ZG that are responsible for the production of aldosterone, because 18-hydroxylase and 18-hydroxysteroid dehydrogenase (18-OHSDH), the mitochondrial enzymes necessary for conversion of corticosterone to aldosterone, are found there.

The bulk of the adrenal cortex comprises the ZF, which consists of regular columns of large cells, laden with cholesterol. They are commonly referred to as 'clear' cells because, under the light microscope, they appear vacuolated when their cholesterol content has been removed by xylene in the fixing and staining procedures.

The third zone (ZR) consists of somewhat smaller, more 'compact' cells. Both this type, and the cells of the ZF, are responsible for the biosynthesis of corticosteroids, androgens and oestrogens from cholesterol

obtained from the adrenal blood supply, but it appears that the latter
cell type only actively synthesises steroids in response to corticotrophin. Indeed, it has been shown that stimulation by ACTH results
in a change of 'clear' cells in the ZF to 'compact' cells of the ZR, so
that there is a marked widening of the latter zone (Figure 3.3).

Biosynthesis of the Corticosteroids

The classical work of Hechter & Pincus in the early 1950s using cow
adrenal led to the belief that progesterone played a key role in the
biosynthesis of all the corticosteroids. Thus, pregnenolone was found to
be converted first to progesterone, as one example of the conversion
of a 5-ene-3β-hydroxysteroid to a 4-en-3-oxosteroid. Several others are
encountered in steroid biosynthetic pathways, notably 17α-hydroxy-
pregnenolone→17α-hydroxyprogesterone, dehydroepiandrosterone→
4-androstenedione and 5-androstenediol→testosterone. These last two
reactions occur in androgen biosynthesis and will be discussed later.
The transformations are carried out by means of a 5-ene-3β-hydroxy-
steroid dehydrogenase (5-ene-3β-OHSDH) and a steroid isomerase,
which are closely associated and occur in the microsomal fraction of
all adrenal cells, in testis (mainly in the interstitial tissue), in ovary and
in placenta.

Intensive *in vivo* and *in vitro* work a decade ago revealed that, in
contrast to cow adrenals, pregnenolone is the parent steroid for the
corticosteroids and that two pathways exist in human adrenocortical
tissue. The evidence for this was initially derived from incubation
studies in which both pregnenolone and progesterone (one labelled
with ^{14}C and the other with ^{3}H) were used as substrates. Both compounds gave rise to corticosteroids but pregnenolone was converted
predominantly to the 17-hydroxylated compounds, 11-deoxycortisol,
cortisol and cortisone, whereas progesterone gave rise mainly to the
17-deoxycorticoids, 11-deoxycorticosterone (DOC), corticosterone and
aldosterone. Figure 3.4 shows the two pathways. One involves the
17-hydroxylation of pregnenolone followed by conversion to
17α-hydroxyprogesterone by means of the 5-ene-3β-OHSDH and
isomerase enzyme system. 21-Hydroxylation occurs next, yielding
11-deoxycortisol. This series of reactions occurs in the microsomal
fraction of adrenal cells but the 11-deoxycortisol must then be trans-
ported into the mitochondria for the final conversion to cortisol,
because the 11β-hydroxylase, requiring NADPH and O_2, is bound to
the inner membrane. When cortisol and corticosterone pass back
into the endoplasmic reticulum, the enzyme 11β-hydroxysteroid

dehydrogenase is encountered and this catalyses the reversible conversion to cortisone and 11-dehydrocorticosterone, respectively.

The second pathway involves the conversion of pregnenolone into progesterone. In the adrenals of man this seems to be of minor importance and helps to explain the smaller amounts of 17-deoxy-corticoids, such as corticosterone, formed from pregnenolone. Progesterone is then hydroxylated at C-21 to yield DOC but the hydroxylation at C-11β to give corticosterone must be accomplished in the mitochondria, as indicated above. Aldosterone is finally produced by means of the intramitochondrial 18-hydroxylase and 18-OHSDH.

Biosynthesis of the Androgens

Although evidence exists for the formation of androgens in semini-ferous tubules, the major site is the interstitial tissue. Smaller amounts are produced by the adrenals in the cells of the ZF and ZR (adrenal androgens) and in the ovaries. As a result of a great number of *in vivo* and *in vitro* studies, two pathways have been discovered for androgen biosynthesis from pregnenolone. One of these involves 5-ene-3β-hydroxysteroid metabolites such as 17α-hydroxypregnenolone and DHA, and is called the '5-ene-3β-hydroxy' pathway; the other involves 4-en-3-oxosteroid metabolites such as progesterone and 17α-hydroxy-progesterone, and is called the '4-en-3-oxo' pathway (Figure 3.5). These are still sometimes referred to as the 'Δ^5' and 'Δ^4' pathways, respec-tively, to indicate the positions of unsaturation in the relevant intermediates. Now that this designation has been dropped from steroid nomenclature in favour of 5-ene and 4-ene, the terms Δ^5 and Δ^4 are not much used.

Figure 3.5 shows that pregnenolone is the parent compound for androgen biosynthesis. One pathway whereby this can be metabolised is by hydroxylation at C-17, after which the side-chain is removed oxidatively as acetate by means of the C-17,20 lyase, to produce DHA. This lyase, together with the 17α-hydroxylase, is tightly bound to the endoplasmic reticulum of androgen-producing tissues and requires NADPH and molecular oxygen for activity. DHA can then be meta-bolised in two ways: (1) to 5-androstene-3β,17β-diol by means of the microsomal 17β-hydroxysteroid dehydrogenase, and thence to testo-sterone by means of the 5-en-3β-OHSDH and steroid isomerase; or (2) to 4-androstenedione and thence to testosterone. It appears that, in human adrenals only, the conversion of DHA to 4-androstenedione is of relatively minor importance.

Figure 3.4: Biosynthetic Pathways of Corticosteroids

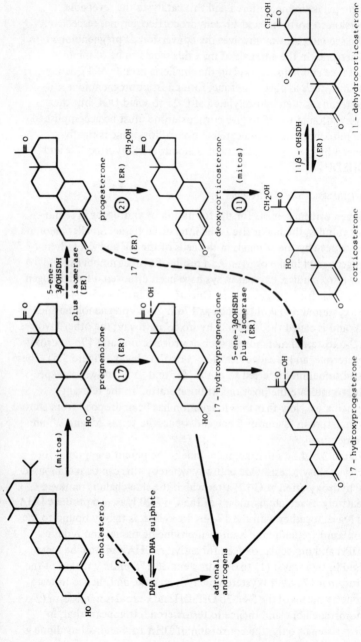

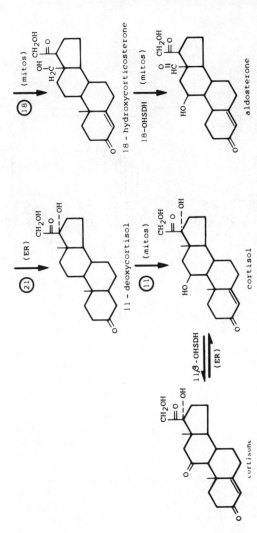

Abbreviations: mitos, mitochondria; ER, endoplasmic reticulum; OHDSH, hydroxysteroid dehydrogenase; (7) indicates the position of hydroxylation; → indicates a reaction; --→ indicates a minor pathway in the human adrenal cortex; $\xrightarrow{?}$ indicates a possible reaction.

Figure 3.5:
Biosynthetic Pathways of
Androgens (abbreviations as
in Figure 3.4)

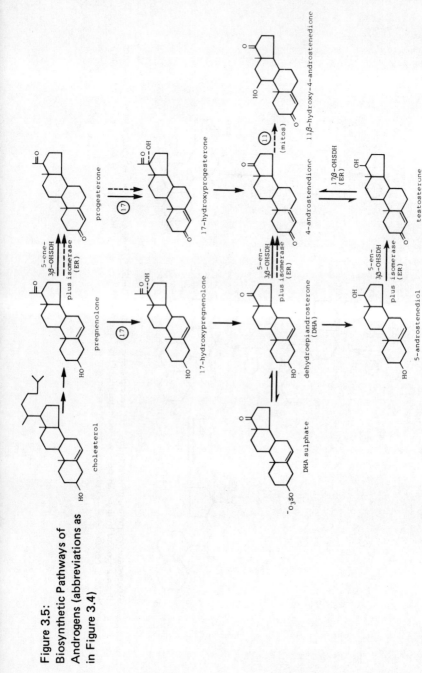

The 4-en-3-oxosteroid pathway consists of the initial conversion of pregnenolone to progesterone, catalysed by the 5-en-3β-OHSDH-isomerase; as in the case of DHA above, this reaction is of minor importance in human adrenals. Next, progesterone is 17α-hydroxylated and the side-chain removed, resulting in the formation of 4-androstenedione. The final conversion to the potent androgen, testosterone, is catalysed by the 17β-OHSDH. Testosterone can be reduced in ring A, by the 5α-reductase found in testis, skin and salivary glands, to form 5α-dihydrotestosterone (5α-DHT). In androgen target tissues, such as prostate, however, 5α-DHT is formed in the cytoplasm and also in the nucleus, the latter reduction being characteristic for such tissues. It is commonly thought that 5α-DHT may be the active form of testosterone and that it is the binding of 5α-DHT to the DNA of androgen-dependent tissues that subsequently results in the manifestation of physiological and biochemical reactions (see Chapter 4). 5α-DHT is metabolised further in the cytoplasm to 5α-androstane-3α,17β- and 3β,17β-diols.

Biosynthesis of Adrenal Androgens. The formation of C_{19} steroids in the adrenals has been alluded to already (see also Figure 3.4). Evidence from *in vitro* and *in vivo* experiments in numerous species has shown that both pathways of androgen biosynthesis occur. However, being in adrenal tissue, the action of the 11β-hydroxylase is also encountered, and this brings about the conversion of 4-androstenedione to 11β-hydroxy-4-androstenedione. The rate of 11β-hydroxylation is only about 30 per cent that of deoxycorticosterone, so that this is considered to be of relatively minor importance. It should be noted that 11β-hydroxy-4-androstenedione is formed as a metabolite of cortisol when its side-chain is cleaved oxidatively (see Chapter 5).

Formation of Steroid Sulphates. In the cytosol of adrenal (ZR and ZF), testis, ovary, liver and foetal tissues, sulphokinases are found, which catalyse the conversion of steroids to steroid sulphates, in the presence of ATP. The enzymes act most efficiently with 5-ene-3β-hydroxysteroids (such as DHA) as substrates. Since the early 1960s, numerous steroid sulphates have been isolated and it has been shown that they can be metabolised as esters without prior hydrolysis of the sulphate moiety. Thus, steroid sulphate pathways have been proposed, which parallel those of the free unesterified steroids, viz., cholesterol sulphate $\rightarrow$ pregnenolone sulphate $\rightarrow$ 17α-hydroxypregnenolone sulphate $\rightarrow$ DHA sulphate $\rightarrow$ 5-androstenediol sulphate. Such pathways, however, are usually of minor importance compared with free steroid pathways.

The physiological significance of steroid sulphates is still not fully understood but it seems possible that DHA sulphate and 5-androstenediol sulphate represent circulating stores of potential androgens, because sulphatases exist which can convert these conjugates to the free steroids and these, in turn, can be transformed into 4-androstenedione and testosterone, respectively (Figure 3.5). DHA sulphate is also especially important in the biosynthesis of oestrogens (see Chapter 7).

Biosynthesis of the Oestrogens

The ovaries are the main source of oestrogens in pre-menopausal women. Both the follicular tissue and the corpora lutea are responsible for the biosynthesis of oestradiol-17β, oestrone and oestriol. As in the testes and the adrenals, the parent compound, cholesterol, is converted to pregnenolone and this subsequently gives rise to 4-androstenedione and testosterone by way of the '4-en-3-oxo' and '5-ene-3β-hydroxy' pathways. Ovarian tissue, however, contains a series of enzymes which is responsible for the conversion of these androgens to oestrogens. 4-Androstenedione and testosterone are 19-hydroxylated first (microsomal 19-hydroxylase); the 19-hydroxyl groups are then oxidised to aldehyde groups (microsomal 19-hydroxysteroid dehydrogenase) and, finally, these are removed as methanal (microsomal C-10,19 lyase). Spontaneous rearrangement results in an aromatic ring A (Figure 3.6), the final products being oestradiol-17β from testosterone and oestrone from 4-androstenedione. The microsomal 16α-hydroxylase of ovary, testis and foetal liver catalyses the conversion of oestradiol-17β into oestriol. All four enzymes involved in oestrogen biosynthesis require NADPH and oxygen for activity and are cytochrome P-450-dependent.

Oestrogens are also produced from other sources. For example, the adrenals synthesise oestrone, although the small quantities formed are relatively unimportant. The testes also produce oestrogen in much higher quantities than was at one time thought. Recent evidence indicates that, in some men, up to 30 per cent of the total oestrogen is formed here. Other recent work has revealed that peripheral tissues have the ability to utilise plasma 4-androstenedione and testosterone to synthesise oestrogens in both men and women. In post-menopausal women, most of the oestrogen produced comes from plasma 4-androstenedione.

The foeto-placental unit in pregnancy is also, of course, responsible for oestrogen production, but this will be considered in Chapter 7.

Figure 3.6: Biosynthetic Pathways of Oestrogens (abbreviations as in Figure 3.4)

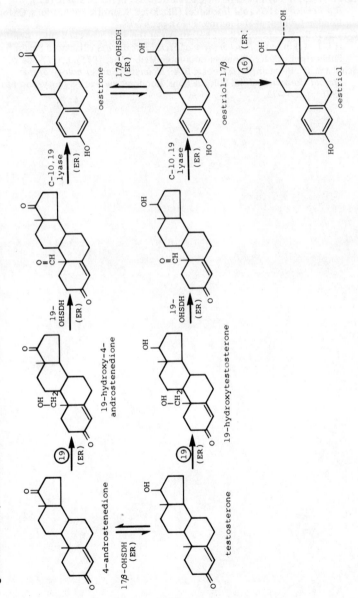

References

Gower, D.B., 'Biosynthesis of the Corticosteroids', in H.L.J. Makin (ed.), *Biochemistry of Steroid Hormones* (Blackwell Scientific Publications, Oxford-London-Edinburgh-Melbourne, 1975), pp. 47-75.

Gower, D.B., & Fotherby, K., 'Biosynthesis of the Androgens and Oestrogens', in H.L.J. Makin (ed.), *Biochemistry of Steroid Hormones* (Blackwell Scientific Publications, Oxford-London-Edinburgh-Melbourne, 1975), pp. 77-104.

Schulster, D., Burstein, S., & Cooke, B.A., *Molecular Endocrinology of the Steroid Hormones* (John Wiley & Sons, London-New York-Sydney-Toronto, 1976), pp. 44-72.

4 MECHANISM OF ACTION

The physiological and biochemical actions of corticosteroids, androgens and oestrogens have been described in Chapter 2. One of the great problems is to explain how a single steroid can bring about such numerous and diverse actions. The glucocorticoids, for example, exert powerful effects on glucose and nitrogen metabolism by inducing some of the enzymes involved in gluconeogenesis, but they also affect collagen synthesis and fibroblast formation.

In the early 1960s, Jacob and Monod published a theory to explain the induction of enzymes in bacteria, and current ideas about the way in which steroid hormones act in animal systems are based on this earlier work. Figure 4.1 shows the Jacob-Monod theory, which postulates the synthesis of a *repressor* protein whose overall reaction is to prevent the synthesis of other proteins (enzymes). In the presence of the *inducer*, however (in this case, the steroid), the configuration of the repressor is altered by reacting with the inducer, thereby relieving its inhibitory effects on specific enzyme synthesis. In animal and human systems, the inducer must enter the cell, find its way to the nucleus and then interact with the DNA. These steps are complex, and it is only during the past fifteen to twenty years that there have been any clues as to how they might occur. A considerable advance was made in 1962, when the work of Jensen and Jacobsen distinguished between target and non-target tissues. These workers injected [^{3}H] oestradiol-17β subcutaneously into immature rats and found that, although there was an initial rapid uptake of radioactivity into muscle, blood, kidney and liver, the high levels were not maintained but dropped to quite low values by some sixteen hours after the injection. In contrast, vagina and uterus retained labelled oestadiol-17β for much longer periods. Furthermore, these responsive (or target) tissues retained their radio-activity largely as oestradiol-17β, while in the non-responsive (or non-target) tissues, this was converted to various metabolites, some being free and some conjugated, but all with lower oestrogenic activity. Further work showed that, within a short time after administration, the steroid was found to be concentrated in the nuclei of target tissue cells. Thus, from the results of these and other experiments, it was realised that only some tissues were responsive to steroid hormones and that the latter probably exerted their primary effects on the nucleus

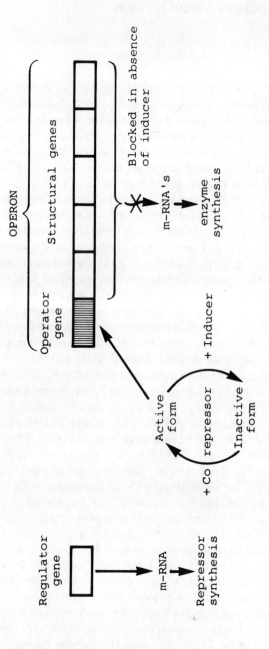

Figure 4.1: Suggested Scheme for the Mechanism of Enzyme Induction

(i.e., probably on the nuclear chromatin).

Investigations were pursued by a number of researchers who used actinomycin D, cycloheximide and puromycin (which inhibit protein synthesis at different stages) and which were in turn shown to inhibit the effects of various steroids. Actinomycin D inhibits m-RNA synthesis by binding to guanosine residues of DNA, while cycloheximide and puromycin block protein synthesis at later stages. Cycloheximide prevents transfer of amino acids from t-RNA to the growing polypeptide chain, while puromycin prematurely terminates the assembly of polypeptides. Thus, these results indicated that the effects of steroids were mediated through m-RNA and protein synthesis.

The next question was how the active steroids could be taken up by target cells and then find their way to the nucleus, where they could exert their effects on m-RNA synthesis. Partial answers to this question came with the isolation of special protein molecules (so-called 'receptors') from the cytoplasm of target tissues which specifically bind the appropriate steroids. Thus, receptors for oestradiol-17β and progesterone were discovered in vagina and uterus and receptors to androgens were found in androgen-responsive tissues like the prostate and seminal vesicles. Many such cytoplasmic receptors have now been characterised. They are usually protein in nature, although some contain a carbohydrate or lipid component. Once the steroid has entered the target cell it binds with the cytoplasmic receptors. The binding has been found to be of the high-affinity, low-capacity type, the receptors being easily saturated. The steroid-receptor complex (Figure 4.2) then moves to the nucleus — the second step in the 'two-step' process. This transference to the nucleus is temperature-dependent and occurs only slowly at 4°C but rapidly at 37°C.

For oestradiol-17β, the available evidence suggests that initial cytoplasmic binding occurs to a protein which sediments at 4S in the ultracentrifuge, but the nuclear component is a different 5S protein. Whether the 4S protein in the cytosol 'hands over' the steroid to the 5S receptor in the nucleus or whether the 5S receptor is a modified 4S protein is not yet clear; neither is the interaction of the steroid and the nuclear chromatin properly understood. O'Malley and Schrader (1976), however, have reviewed some recent experiments to indicate which part of the DNA is involved in binding. They have worked with progesterone in the chick oviduct and have shown that the receptor consists of two sub-units, A and B, each of which possesses a site for binding one molecule of steroid. It is the B sub-unit which binds to the AP$_3$ fraction of the non-histone proteins of the chromatin. The A

Figure 4.2: Suggested Mechanism for the Stimulating Effect of Oestradiol-17β on Protein Synthesis in Target Tissues. R_c denotes a cytoplasmic oestradiol-17β receptor

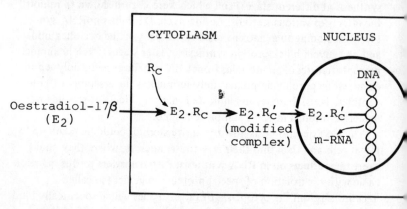

Figure 4.3: Scheme for the Effects of Androgens on Protein Synthesis in Target Tissues. R_c and R_N denote cytoplasmic and nuclear receptors, 5α-DHT denotes 5α-dihydrotestosterone and OHSDH, hydroxysteroid dehydrogenase

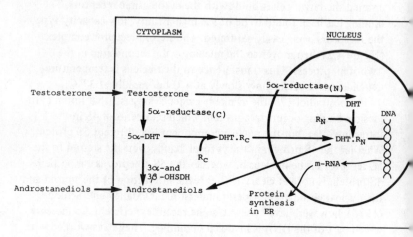

sub-unit only binds directly to the DNA and cannot associate with the chromatin. Thus, it is conceivable that the dimer dissociates after the B sub-unit has been bound to the protein. In binding to the non-histone fraction, it is thought that the steroid-A sub-unit complex alters an inactive initiation site so that RNA polymerase can occupy the site. Alternatively, it may be that a hitherto concealed site is revealed. There is certainly abundant evidence that the activity of RNA polymerase increases markedly in target tissues in response to steroid. Thus, a specific segment of DNA, once revealed by the steroid-A sub-unit complex, can be transcribed and the m-RNA used in the synthesis of spcific proteins.

The physiological actions of testosterone depend on its being reduced to 5α-dihydrotestosterone (5α-DHT) in the cytoplasm by means of the 5α-reductase. This reduction also occurs in the nucleus and is a characteristic feature of some androgen-responsive tissues. It is thought that testosterone first enters the cytoplasm of the target cell and is there reduced to 5α-DHT (Figure 4.3), which is bound specifically to receptors (R_c). By a temperature-dependent process, translocation to the nucleus then takes place where the 5α-DHT is transferred to a nuclear receptor (R_N). Interaction with the DNA results in the synthesis of m-RNA and hence in specific protein synthesis. Alternatively, testosterone may pass straight to the nucleus where 5α-DHT formation will occur by the nuclear 5α-reductase. Inactivation probably takes place in the cytoplasm by further reduction to 5α-androstane-3α,17β-diol and 5α-androstane-3β,17β-diol through the action of 3α- and 3β-hydroxysteroid dehydrogenases. Both these compounds possess less androgenic potency than 5α-DHT.

In a similar way, testosterone is thought to be converted to oestrogen in hypothalamic/pituitary tissue prior to exerting its 'feedback' effects (see Chapter 6). The possibility that many steroid hormones circulating in plasma may require metabolic alteration before exerting effects on target tissues must not be forgotten. Our knowledge of the precise way in which steroid hormones act is still therefore limited and much work continues in efforts to elucidate more precisely how these small molecules exert such profound and diverse effects.

Reference

O'Malley, B.W., & Schrader, W.T., 'The Receptors of Steroid Hormones', *Scientific American* (1976), vol. 234, pp. 32-43.

5 CATABOLISM AND CONJUGATION

Various hormones are secreted by the adrenals and gonads into the peripheral circulation. Numerous reactions subsequently occur, notably in the liver and to some extent in the kidneys, which inactivate the physiologically-active steroids. These reactions are mainly, though not exclusively, reductive in nature and tend to render the molecules more polar. Thus, various steroids, such as cortisol, testosterone and oestradiol-17β, have finite biological half-lives in the peripheral circulation, and the plasma concentration at a particular time depends (a) on the rate of secretion of the steroid from the tissues in which it has been synthesised and (b) on the rate at which it is irreversibly removed by catabolic processes — i.e., the 'metabolic clearance rate'. The inactivated metabolites are then converted by the process of conjugation to sulphate esters or glucuronides, so that the lipophilic steroids are thereby converted into more water-soluble conjugates, which can be excreted in the urine.

Four main pathways are involved in the catabolism of steroid hormones:

(1) reduction of the double bond at C-4, together with reduction of the oxo group at C-3 to a secondary alcoholic group;
(2) reduction of the oxo group at C-20 to a secondary alcoholic group;
(3) oxidation of a 17β-hydroxyl group; and
(4) further hydroxylation at various points in the steroid nucleus.

These methods will be illustrated by reference to the catabolism of C_{21}, C_{19} and C_{18} steroids.

The Corticosteroids

As described in Chapter 2, this group of steroids contains the 4-en-3-oxo configuration. Catabolism (method 1) takes place first by reduction in the A-ring by means of two enzymes, a microsomal 4-ene-5α-reductase and a soluble 4-ene-5β-reductase, which require NADPH. Secondly, reduction at C-3 occurs by means of the 3α- and 3β-hydroxysteroid dehydrogenases, microsomal enzymes which require NADH or NADPH for activity. In theory, therefore, a corticosteroid such as

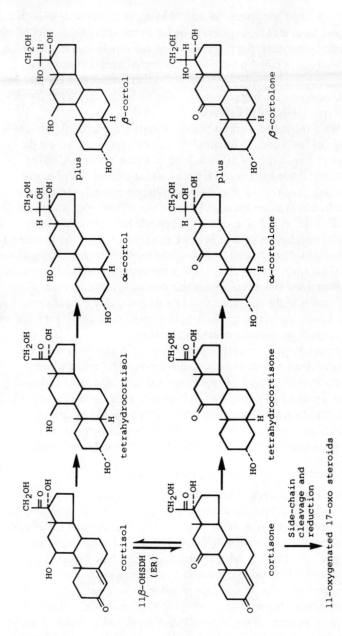

Figure 5.1: Abbreviated Catabolic Pathways of Cortisol and Cortisone

cortisol could give rise to 3α- and 3β-hydroxy compounds of both the 5α and 5β series but, in practice, owing to the relative activities of the reductive enzymes, the predominant metabolite in man is tetrahydro-cortisol (or tetrahydro F,THF) – the 3α,5β-isomer (Figure 5.1). Cortisone can be readily reduced at C-11 to cortisol (see Chapter 3) and the corresponding reduced metabolite in this case is tetrahydro-cortisone (tetrahydro E,THE).

Since the corticosteroids possess an oxo group at C-20, this is also available for reduction (method 2). The enzymes involved are the cyto-plasmic 20α- and 20β-OHSDHs, both of which prefer NADPH as cofactor; the reduction of THF results in the formation of α- and β-cortols (Figure 5.1). The corresponding compounds formed from tetrahydrocortisone are α- and β-cortolones. These six compounds (THF, THE, α- and β-cortols, α- and β-cortolones), together with similar metabolites derived from other corticosteroids, are excreted as glucuronides (see below), and comprise the bulk of the 17-oxogenic steroids. These are so called because the method for their estimation in urine involves a glycol-fission reaction which results in the conversion of the side-chain to a 17-oxo group (the oxogenic reaction). The 17-oxo steroids thus formed can then be estimated by the Zimmer-mann reaction (alkaline m-dinitrobenzene).

About 10 per cent of 17-hydroxylated corticosteroids can be metabolised by oxidative side-chain cleavage, the products being 17-oxosteroids. If an 11-oxygen function is present, as in cortisol, 11-oxygenated 17-oxosteroids are formed. Thus, cortisol would initially yield 11β-hydroxy-4-androstenedione (Figure 5.1) and this, on reduction, would lead to two 11-hydroxylated 17-oxosteroids. Corresponding 11-oxo-17-oxosteroids are obtained from cortisone.

Progesterone and 17α-Hydroxyprogesterone

Both these C_{21} steroids are metabolised by reductive methods 1 and 2, although the catabolism differs depending on the tissue concerned. In ovary and uterus, reduction of progesterone occurs at C-20 (method 2) to give the progestationally active 20α and 20β reduced progesterones (Figure 5.2). Further reduction takes place in these tissues as well as in liver at ring A and at C-3 (method 1) and results in a series of six pregnanediols. The most important of these is 5β-pregnane-3α,20α-diol, which is excreted in urine, conjugated as glucuronide, and accounts for 10 to 30 per cent of the metabolites of progesterone. Similar reactions occur for 17α-hydroxyprogesterone, yielding, principally, 5β-pregnane-3α,17α,20α-triol (pregnanetriol).

Figure 5.2: Abbreviated Catabolic Pathways of Progesterone and 17α-Hydroxyprogesterone

progesterone

Method 1

Method 2

pregnanediol
(5β-pregnane-3α, 20α-diol)

17α-hydroxyprogesterone

Method 1

Method 2

pregnanetriol
(5β-pregnane-3α,17α,20α-triol)

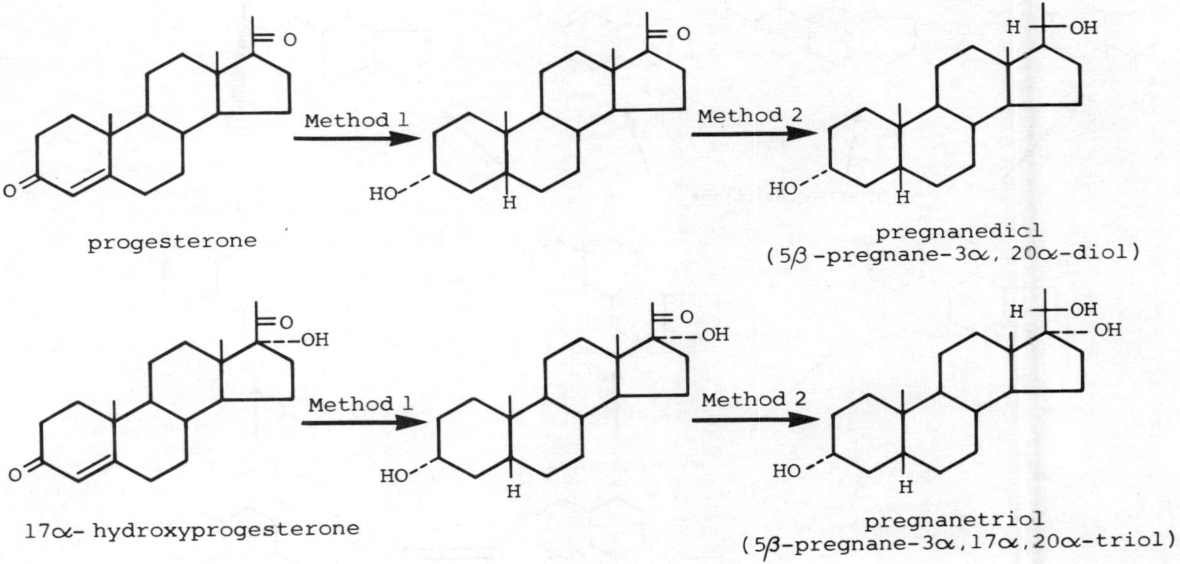

Figure 5.3: Abbreviated Catabolic Pathways of Testosterone

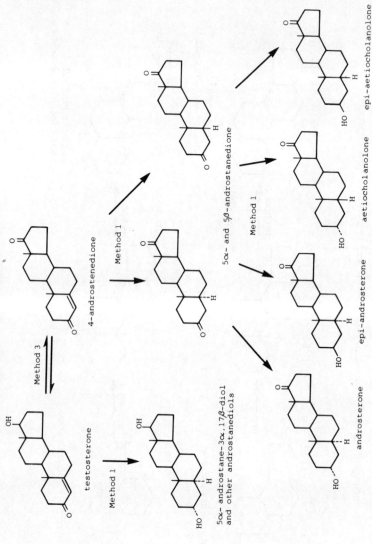

The Androgens

Testosterone loses some 80 per cent of its androgenic potency as oxidation of its 17β-hydroxyl group to a 17-oxo group (4-androstenedione) occurs (method 3). Further reduction (method 1) of this compound leads first to the ring A-saturated steroids, 5α and 5β-androstane-3,17-diones (Figure 5.3). Reduction at C-3 leads to the formation of four isomeric 17-oxosteroids, androsterone (3α, 5α-), aetiocholanolone (3α,5β-), epi-androsterone (3β,5α-) and epi-aetiocholanolone (3β,5β-). It should be noted, however, that the 3β-hydroxy compounds occur in only small quantities. These are excreted, conjugated partly as sulphates and partly as glucuronides. In a similar way, testosterone is reduced (method 1) but, owing to the presence of the 17β-hydroxyl group, the metabolites are isomeric androstanediols, principally 5α- and 5β-androstane-3α,17β-diols. 11-Hydroxy- and 11-oxo-4-androstenediones, which are produced in the adrenals and peripheral tissues by side-chain cleavage of cortisol and cortisone, respectively (see above), suffer a similar fate to that of 4-androstenedione, yielding 11-oxygenated 17-oxosteroids.

As seen in Chapter 3, the adrenals produce DHAS in large quantities and this, together with DHA, is reduced in the liver, by means of the 17β-OHSDH, to 5-androstenediol and its sulphate. The former is conjugated with glucuronic acid before being excreted, while the sulphate is excreted intact. The urine also contains DHAS and, since this is a 17-oxosteroid, it can be measured after conjugate hydrolysis, along with androsterone and its isomers, by the Zimmerman reaction. Table 5.1 summarises the quantities of steroid metabolites excreted in human urine.

The Oestrogens

The oxidation (method 3) of oestradiol-17β to oestrone has been referred to already in Chapter 2, and by this reaction some oestrogenic potency is lost. Further hydroxylation or ketone formation at various positions in the molecule result in loss of more oestrogenicity (Figure 5.4). The most important reaction is that of 16α-hydroxylation, leading to oestriol (see Chapter 7), but hydroxylation can also occur at C-2, C-4, C-6α and 6β, C-7α, C-14α, C-15α, C-16β and C-18. Some twenty oestrogens can thus be found in human urine, conjugated as glucuronides and sulphates. Some of the very polar 6- or 7-oxygenated derivatives (e.g., 6-hydroxyoestriol) appear to be sufficiently water-soluble to occur as free steroids.

Table 5.1: Values for the Urinary Excretion of Some Steroids in Healthy Men and Women

	MEN			WOMEN	
	mg/24 h	μmoles/24 h		mg/24 h	μmoles/24 h
17-oxosteroids	5-20	13-66		5-15	11-40
17-oxogenic steroids	7-20	15-80		5-15	15-70
Testosterone	0.22	0.77		0.02	0.07
Pregnanediol	0.6	0-4.4	FP[a]	0.9	0-5.2
			LP	2.6	5.2-26.0
			P	45	160
Pregnanetriol	1.6	0-10.7	FP	0.35	0-7.3
			LP	0.9	
Total oestrogens	0.006	0-0.04	FP	0.006	0.02-0.155
			LP	0.032	0.045-0.29
Oestradiol-17β	0.0008	0-0.003	FP	0.002	0.007
			LP	0.004	0.012
			P	0.1-1.0	0.35-3.5
Oestrone	0.002	0-0.013	FP	0.004	0.012
			LP	0.01	0.035
			P	0.01-1.0	0.035-3.5
Oestriol	0.003	0-0.02	FP	0.005	0.017
			LP	0.016	0.056
			P	35.0	123.0

a. Notation: FP, follicular phase; LP, luteal phase; P, pregnancy, week 39.

Figure 5.4: Catabolism of Oestrogens

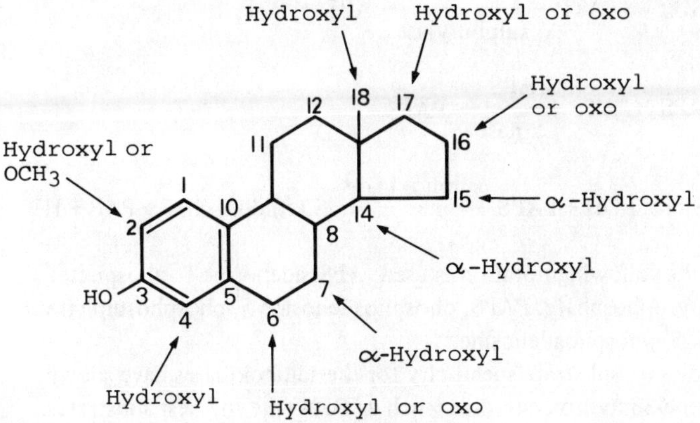

Steroid Conjugation

Glucuronides. These conjugates are formed by reaction of the steroid metabolite with uridine diphosphoglucuronic acid (UDPGA) in the presence of glucuronyl transferases, which are found in liver microsomal fraction. Thus

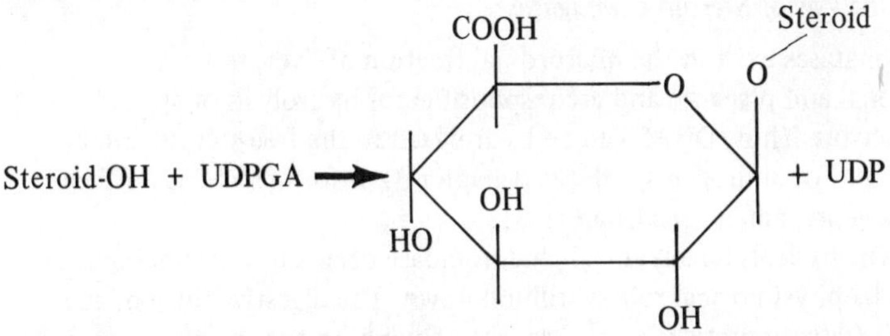

Steroid-OH + UDPGA $\longrightarrow$ + UDP

where UDP denotes uridine diphosphate.

Glucuronides are readily excreted by the kidneys, the clearance rate approximating that of the glomerular filtration rate.

Sulphates. Sulphokinases occur in the cytosol of cells of the liver, testis, adrenals (zona reticularis and fasciculata, but not zona glomerulosa) and foetal tissues. These enzymes catalyse the reaction between a steroid and 'active' sulphate (phosphoadenosine-5'-phosphosulphate); magnesium ions are necessary for activity. The reaction occurs in three stages:

$$(1) \quad SO_4^{2-} + ATP \xrightarrow[\text{sulphurylase}]{ATP} APS + P-P_i$$

$$(2) \quad APS + ATP \xrightarrow[\text{kinase}]{APS} PAPS$$

$$(3) \quad \text{Steroid-OH} + PAPS \xrightarrow{\text{sulphokinase}} \text{Steroid-O}-SO_3^- + PAP + H^+$$

where the following notation is used: APS, adenosine-5′-phosphate; P–P$_i$, pyrophosphate; PAPS, phosphoadenosine-5′-phosphosulphate; PAP, 3′,5′-phosphoadenosine.

Studies on substrate specificity for the sulphokinases have shown that 5-ene-3β-hydroxysteroids (such as DHA) are the best substrates. The ease of sulphation of the corresponding ring-B reduced compounds (5β-series) is less. This series, in turn, is more easily sulphated than the 5α-series. If other hydroxyl groups are present in the molecule, it is the hydroxyl at C-3 that is preferentially sulphated. The renal clearance of steroid sulphates is much lower than that of glucuronides, being only about 10 per cent of the glomerular filtration rate.

Hydrolysis of Steroid Conjugates

Sulphatases exist in the microsomal fraction of liver, testis, ovary, adrenal and placenta and are responsible for hydrolysis of steroid sulphates. Thus, DHAS can be hydrolysed to the free steroid and be utilised for androgen synthesis (Chapter 3) or for oestrogen synthesis during pregnancy (see Chapter 7).

The hydrolytic enzyme β-glucuronidase occurs in intestinal mucosa but its physiological role is still unknown. The digestive juice of the snail *Helix pomatia* is a good source of sulphatases and of β-glucuronidase and such preparations, which are commercially available, are of great value in hydrolysing urinary steroid conjugates to the free steroids *in vitro*. After solvent extraction, these can be separated and estimated, commonly by gas-liquid chromatography or high pressure liquid chromatography. If estimation of oestrogens is required, use is made of the solubility of these steroids in sodium hydroxide solution, so that they can be separated from other steroids which are also soluble in ether. Subsequent acidification and re-extraction results in a total oestrogen extract. These can be estimated in pregnancy urine as total oestrogen (mainly oestriol) using the Köber reaction (a phenol-concentrated sulphuric acid), which gives a yellow colour that turns red on dilution

with water. Alternatively the individual oestrogens can be separated
and estimated using gas-liquid chromatography. Oestrogens in non-
pregnant women's urine, or in men, are generally estimated using
radioimmunoassay or combined gas chromatography-mass specto-
metry. Table 5.1 summarises the quantities of oestrogens excreted in
human urine.

6 OCCURRENCE IN HUMAN BLOOD PLASMA AND CONTROL OF STEROID SECRETION

In general, a high proportion of the steroid hormones present in plasma is bound to plasma proteins — specifically to globulins and non-specifically to albumin. This means that only a proportion of the steroids (ranging from 1-2 per cent for androgens and 6 per cent for cortisol to 40 per cent for aldosterone) circulates in the free, unbound form. Many years ago, it was suggested that plasma proteins 'buffered' steroid hormones, and more recent research has largely confirmed this view, because it is only the free fraction of steroids in plasma that appears to be physiologically active. Thus, it is known, for example, that androgen administration decreases the concentration of the plasma globulin that binds testosterone, while oestrogen administration increases the globulin concentration, thereby altering, in each case, the level of metabolically-active, free testosterone.

Corticosteroids in Plasma

Table 6.1 summarises the various corticosteroids with their concentrations that are found in human plasma. As indicated above, approximately 94 per cent of glucocorticoids are protein-bound, two proteins being involved. The more important is cortisol-binding globulin (CBG) or transcortin, which has high affinity and low capacity and binds about 80 per cent of plasma cortisol. In spite of its name, CBG is not specific for cortisol but also binds corticosterone and progesterone. During oestrogen therapy, in pregnant women or in women taking the steroidal oral pill, the concentration of CBG increases, thus transiently reducing the amount of physiologically active, free, plasma cortisol. This is particularly relevant in late pregnancy when, despite increased levels of total plasma cortisol, no symptoms of hyperadrenalism occur as a result of increased plasma CBG concentrations.

The remaining bound cortisol, approximately 15 per cent, is bound to albumin which shows low-affinity, high-capacity binding characteristics. For aldosterone, there is no specific binding globulin but 60 per cent is bound to albumin.

Table 6.1: Concentrations of Some Steroid Hormones in the Plasma of Healthy Men and Women

	MEN		WOMEN		
	nmol/litre	ng/100 ml		nmol/litre	ng/100 ml
Cortisol (at 9.00 a.m.)	420	16000		420	16000
Corticosteroids[a] (at 9.00 a.m.)	158-683	6000-26000			
(at midnight)	210	8000			
Aldosterone (normal Na+-ion intake)					
supine	0.1-0.33	3.5-11.5			
ambulant	0.2-0.66	7-23			
Progesterone	0.95	30	FP[b]	4.4	140
			LP	33	1050
			P	555	17500
17-OH-progesterone	3	90	FP	1.2	40
			LP	5	170
			P	18	600
Testosterone	9-24	700		1.7	50
Testosterone glucuronide	6.5	300			
DHA sulphate	3900	143000		2170	80000
DHA	17	500		17	500
Androsterone sulphate	1220	45000		540	20000
Androsterone	5.5	160		2.4	70
Aetiocholanolone	1.2	35		1.4	40
Oestrone	0.13	3.6	FP	0.147	4
			OV	0.55	15
			LP	0.73	20
			P	27.4	750
Oestradiol-17β	0.08	2.3	FP	0.11	3
			OV	2.1	57
			LP	1.46	40
			P	55.0	1500
Oestriol	0.035	1.0	FP	0.07	2
			OV	1.3	37
			P	49	1400

a. Measured by fluorimetry.
b. Notation: FP, follicular phase; OV, ovulatory peak; LP, luteal phase; P, pregnancy, week 39.

Androgens in Plasma

Two plasma proteins are concerned with androgen binding, albumin (non-specifically) and a globulin (specifically). The latter was at one time thought to bind only testosterone and was called testosterone-binding globulin but, since it binds with other steroids possessing a 17β-hydroxyl group such as 5α-dihydrotestosterone and oestradiol-17β, the protein is now designated 'sex hormone-binding globulin' (SHBG). In the case of plasma testosterone in men, some 60 per cent occurs bound to SHBG, 38 per cent to albumin and a mere 2 per cent occurs conjugated as glucuronide. The very weak androgens, such as dehydroepiandrosterone and androsterone, occur largely as their sulphates, loosely bound to plasma albumin. Much smaller quantities exist as unconjugated steroids also loosely bound to albumin. As for CBG mentioned earlier, the concentration of SHBG in plasma varies with androgen or oestrogen administration, the concentration in the plasma of men being half that in the plasma of women, and SHBG has a capacity of up to twice the normal male testosterone content. In addition to the effects of androgens and oestrogens, thyroid hormones increase, while growth hormone decreases the plasma concentration of SHBG.

Plasma levels of androgens are given in Table 6.1.

Progesterone and Oestrogens in Plasma

Progesterone occurs in plasma almost entirely (up to 98 per cent) bound to albumin and CBG, the affinity for the latter being about three times that for cortisol.

The situation as far as the oestrogens is concerned is more complicated. About 66 per cent of the total oestradiol-17β in plasma is unconjugated, while only some 20 per cent of oestrone, and less than 10 per cent of oestriol, occur as the free steroids. Oestriol conjugates are known to include sulphate, glucuronide or mixed sulphate-glucuronide. In contrast, virtually all the conjugated oestrone is present as the sulphate.

Pituitary Hormones and Control of Plasma Cortisol

Corticotrophin (adrenocorticotrophic hormone, ACTH) has long been known to be intimately concerned in the regulation of plasma cortisol levels in man. Human ACTH is a single-chain polypeptide of molecular weight about 4500, containing 39 amino acids. Only the N-terminal 1-24 amino acids are necessary for biological activity, while the others are probably concerned with immunological response. The following events occur in response to increased levels of ACTH: the adrenals increase in size (hyperplasia), adrenal blood flow increases, adrenal cholesterol ester hydrolysis increases, the content of adrenal cholesterol, lipid and ascorbic acid is reduced, biosynthesis of corticosteroids and androgens from cholesterol is increased and both glycogenolysis and glucose metabolism in the adrenals increase. Some of these effects are extremely rapid; for example, in experiments with isolated adrenal cells *in vitro*, the maximum corticosteroid synthesis was attained only three minutes after addition of ACTH. There is good evidence that adenosine-$3',5'$-cyclic monophosphate (c-AMP) is involved because tissue levels of this cyclic nucleotide increase before any increase in steroid biosynthesis is detected. Furthermore, if c-AMP breakdown is inhibited using phosphodiesterase inhibitors like theophylline or caffeine, tissue levels of c-AMP rise and steroid biosynthesis increases even in the absence of ACTH. The evidence suggests that the major site of action of ACTH is between cholesterol and pregnenolone, probably as a result of enhanced binding of cholesterol to cytochrome P-450, which plays a vital role in hydroxylation and side-chain cleavage (see Chapter 3). In addition, the influence of ACTH on cholesterol ester hydrolysis in the adrenal cell increases the cholesterol available for steroid biosynthesis and this is undoubtedly an important factor in the stimulatory effects of the hormone. Stimulatory actions on the adrenal enzymes, 11β-hydroxylase, 18-hydroxylase and 5-ene-3β-OHSDH, have also been described but these are probably of relatively minor importance.

Now that sensitive methods are available for the measurement of plasma ACTH and gonadotrophins, it has been shown that secretion of ACTH by the anterior pituitary does not remain at a constant level throughout a 24-h period, but undergoes a nyctohemeral rhythm, and that plasma levels vary in a pulse-like fashion throughout this period. Thus, mean plasma levels are lowest towards midnight (approximately 0.4 mU/ml or 4 pg/ml) and maximal around 8.00 a.m. (approximately 6 mU/ml or 60 pg/ml). These patterns are reflected in changes in plasma cortisol and androgens, which are lowest in the late evening and maximal between 6.00 a.m. and 8.00 a.m. Patterns are sometimes difficult to discern, but are nevertheless reproducible from day to day and constitute nyctohemeral rhythms (Figures 6.1 and 8.1). Generally, maximal cortisol levels are between 165 and 700 nmol/litre (6.0-25.3 μg/100 ml) with levels falling to a minimum of around 100 nmol/litre (3.6 μg/100 ml).

The secretion of ACTH increases markedly in response to stimula-

Figure 6.1: Changes in Plasma Corticosteroid (upper) and ACTH (lower) Concentrations throughout One 24-h Period in Three Normal Subjects

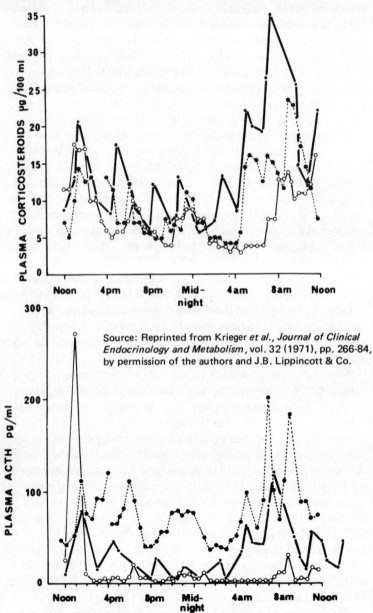

Source: Reprinted from Krieger *et al., Journal of Clinical Endocrinology and Metabolism*, vol. 32 (1971), pp. 266-84, by permission of the authors and J.B. Lippincott & Co.

tion of higher neural areas, as summarised in Figure 6.2. This causes the release of corticotrophin releasing factor (CRF) from the hypothalamus and hence increases ACTH. Such stimuli include surgery (when plasma values increase to 4-12 mU/ml or 40-120 pg/ml), emotional disturbance and infection.

Figure 6.2: Normal Control of Pituitary-adrenal Function in Man

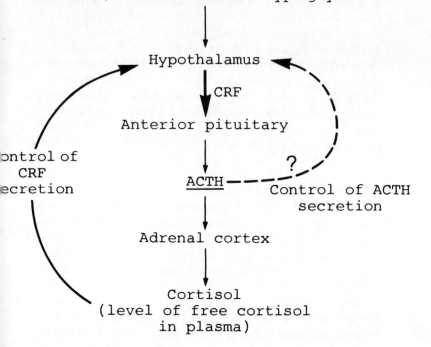

ACTH release is also controlled by plasma cortisol levels in man by a negative feedback mechanism. When plasma cortisol is low, ACTH release is initiated at the level of the hypothalamus, whereas raised plasma cortisol levels inhibit release of CRF and hence of ACTH. A second mechanism may exist whereby plasma levels of ACTH can inhibit anterior pituitary activity.

Control of Aldosterone Biosynthesis

The mechanisms which control the biosynthesis of aldosterone have been studied intensively and, as a result, numerous factors have been discovered which play a part in regulation.

Probably the first control factor to be recognised was that of sodium-ion depletion, which brings about an increase in aldosterone secretion by the cells of the zona glomerulosa of the adrenal cortex via its effect on renal blood flow. It will be recalled from Chapter 2 that a major effect of aldosterone is to conserve sodium ion, and increasing the quantity of this mineralocorticoid would therefore be an effective means of making good the sodium-ion deficiency. In contrast, increasing sodium-ion intake results in reduced aldosterone synthesis and the major control mechanism is through the renin-angiotensin system. The enzyme involved is renin, which is released from the cells of the juxta-glomerula apparatus of the kidney as a result of reduced renal blood flow in response to sodium-ion depletion. The substrate for the enzyme is an α_2-globulin called angiotensinogen, synthesised in the liver (Figure 6.3). From this a decapeptide (angiotensin I) is split off the N-terminal end of the substrate. This biologically inactive compound is transformed into an octapeptide by the cleavage of two amino acid residues from the C-terminal end by means of a 'converting enzyme', found in various tissues, including lung and plasma. This octapeptide is called angiotensin II and, although it is short-lived, exerts powerful effects on aldosterone biosynthesis. The original enzyme renin, which initiates this sequence of events, has a half-life of about fifteen minutes and is degraded by the liver.

Angiotensin II is now known to bind to specific adrenal cortical cell receptors and to stimulate aldosterone synthesis at two sites, one between cholesterol and pregnenolone and the other, at a much later stage in the pathway, between corticosterone and aldosterone, presumably at the 18-hydroxylase/18-hydroxysteroid dehydrogenase steps.

Since angiotensin II stimulates a rapid increase in c-AMP levels in adrenal cells, which precedes the steroidogenic effects, it seems most likely that the cyclic nucleotide is a mediator of the action of

Figure 6.3:
Multi-factorial Control of
Aldosterone Biosynthesis.
⊕ indicates a
stimulatory effect and
⑪ the hydroxylation
position

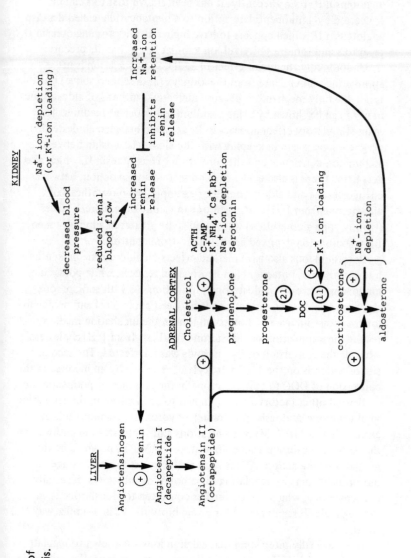

angiotensin II. Fairly recently, it has been shown that this can be converted by aminopeptidase action to a heptapeptide, called des-Asp'-angiotensin II, which appears to have higher affinity for angiotensin II receptors and is more powerful, on a molar basis, than its precursor.

Undoubtedly the major effect of sodium-ion depletion is in stimulating renin release from the kidneys (as described above) but this is not the only mechanism, because increased synthesis of aldosterone *in vitro* can be shown by using a sodium-ion-deficient medium. The main stimulatory effect appears to lie at a step between cholesterol and pregnenolone, again in keeping with the close relationship between sodium-ion deficiency and the formation of angiotensin II, which also acts here. There is also evidence for a second site of action, between corticosterone and aldosterone. For example, the biosynthesis of aldosterone from [^{3}H] corticosterone in canine outer adrenal slices (mainly zona glomerulosa) was found to be greater in adrenals taken from sodium-ion-deprived animals than from controls.

Potassium ions also have marked effects on aldosterone biosynthesis but, in this case, potassium-ion deprivation reduces, while potassium-ion loading increases, aldosterone production. As with sodium ions, there are two sites of action: one is between cholesterol and pregnenolone, because increase of potassium ions in the incubation medium resulted in stimulation of aldosterone synthesis from [^{3}H] cholesterol, whereas the conversion of C_{21} steroids was unaffected. The second site of action is on the 11β-hydroxylase, as shown by an increase in the conversion of DOC to corticosterone in the presence of potassium ions.

Several other factors are also known to be involved in the regulation of aldosterone synthesis. Serotonin (5-hydroxytryptamine) acts at extremely low (10^{-6} M) concentrations and stimulates the pathway at the early cholesterol-pregnenolone stage; c-AMP is known to be the mediator of the action. ACTH is also effective at this early stage but probably acts by regulating the amount of substrates, especially corticosterone, which can be further converted to aldosterone. Prostaglandin E stimulates aldosterone biosynthesis in a similar way to ACTH.

It is especially interesting that calcium ions are known to regulate the actions of ACTH, angiotensin II and potassium ions. If calcium ions are not present, these three factors are without effect. Curiously, calcium ions themselves have little effect on aldosterone biosynthesis either *in vivo* or *in vitro*. However, monovalent ammonium, caesium and rubidium ions all stimulate the pathway, acting between cholesterol and pregnenolone.

In contrast to the above, feedback inhibition by steroids, such as 18-hydroxycorticosterone and aldosterone itself, is recognised at the 18-hydroxylase/18-hydroxysteroid dehydrogenase steps. Thus, the production of aldosterone is tightly controlled by a multifactorial system, summarised in Figure 6.3.

Pituitary Hormones and Plasma Androgen Levels

In addition to ACTH, the anterior pituitary secretes three gonadotrophins: luteinising hormone (LH) or interstitial-cell-stimulating hormone (ICSH), follicle-stimulating hormone (FSH), both from the basophil cells, and prolactin, from the acidophils. Both LH (now called lutotrophin) and FSH (now called follitrophin) are glycoproteins of molecular weights 38 000 and 29 000, respectively, and consist of two polypeptide chains of about 100 amino acids, each linked covalently to a carbohydrate prosthetic group. This comprises some 18-20 per cent of the molecular weight and contains some neutral sugars (mostly mannose, galactose and fucose), hexosamines (mainly N-acetyl-glucosamine, with LH containing N-acetyl galactosamine). Sialic acid is also present to the extent of 5 per cent in FSH and 1 per cent in LH. Studies with neuraminidase indicate that the sialic acid component of FSH is essential for biological activity. By using denaturing agents, it is possible to dissociate both hormones into α- and β-sub-units, which possess little activity and have molecular weights approximately half that of the parent proteins. The α-units are very similar in structure but specificity apparently resides in the β-sub-units.

The third hormone from the human anterior pituitary, prolactin, consists of a single polypeptide chain of 198 amino acids. In mammals it acts mainly as a lactogenic hormone and also influences ovarian steroidogenesis. Although it occurs in the male, its function is not well understood; in the rat, it acts synergistically with LH to stimulate testicular steroidogenesis.

Control of Gonadotrophin Secretion

It is known that gonadotrophins are secreted in a 'pulsatile' manner, similar to that already described for ACTH, the pulses occurring every 30-300 minutes throughout the day and varying in intensity with numerous factors such as age, sex and circulating plasma steroid levels.

At one time it was thought that there were two separate releasing factors secreted by the hypothalamus, one of which stimulated LH secretion and the other stimulated FSH secretion from the anterior pituitary. On the basis of recent evidence, however, it seems that there

Figure 6.4: Hormonal Control of Testicular and Ovarian Steroidogenesis

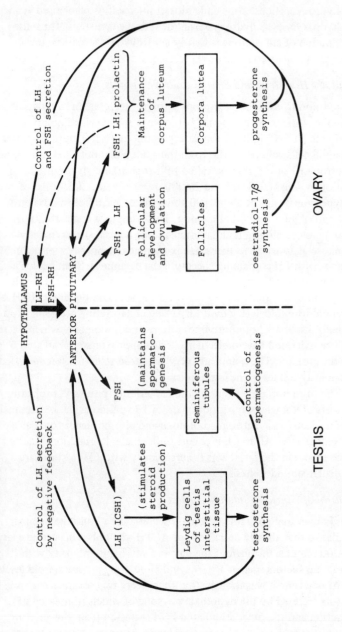

may be only one gonadotrophin-releasing hormone, which is designated
GnRH or, more commonly, FSH-RH/LH-RH. Control of the release of
this hormone from the hypothalamus, and possibly also from the
anterior pituitary and other areas of the brain, occurs by means of
negative feedback from plasma androgens and oestrogens (Figure 6.4).
In contrast, prolactin release is probably controlled partly by an
inhibitory factor, the nature of which has not yet been determined, and
partly by the action of thyrotrophic releasing hormone.

Control of Testicular Function

Both the gonadotrophins, LH and FSH, as well as testosterone, are
necessary for the proper functioning and control of the testis. It was
thought earlier than FSH was the only hormone involved in the control
of spermatogenesis, in the Sertoli cells of the seminiferous tubules.
Current ideas, however, implicate LH as being more important because,
at puberty, this causes stimulation of testosterone formation by the
Leydig cells of the interstitial tissue. Testosterone is known to be at
least partly responsible for the control of spermatogenesis. Thus, the
concentration of testosterone within the testis and the extent of binding to receptor proteins are probably both important factors.

Some androgen formation undoubtedly occurs in the Sertoli cells
but the major processes here are reductive in nature and occur by
means of 20-hydroxysteroid dehydrogenases and 4-en-5α-reductase.
LH is responsible for the stimulation of testicular steroidogenesis from
cholesterol in the Leydig cells (as indicated above) and FSH probably
acts synergistically. Two sites of action are now recognised for LH,
in a similar fashion for the action of ACTH in adrenal steroidogenesis:
(a) by activation of the cytoplasmic testicular cholesterol ester hydro-
lase, so that cholesterol esters are converted into cholesterol; and
(b) by increased mitochondrial side-chain cleavage of hydroxylated
cholesterols, mediated by cytochrome P-450. In addition there is
evidence for increased activity of the 17α-hydroxylase, the C-17,20
lyase, the 4-ene-5α-reductase and, with chronic LH administration,
3β-hydroxysteroid dehydrogenase. As a result, the biosynthesis of
androgens and of all intermediates on the pathway is stimulated.

Plasma Testosterone Levels

In healthy men the average values for testosterone are in the range of
10-31 nmol/litre (290-900 ng/100 ml) of plasma and for women during
the menstrual cycle there is a range of values of 0.5-3.5 nmol/litre
(14-100 ng/100 ml). Although it can be shown that plasma testosterone

Figure 6.5: Changes in Plasma Testosterone Concentrations in 21 Normal Men during One 24-h Period

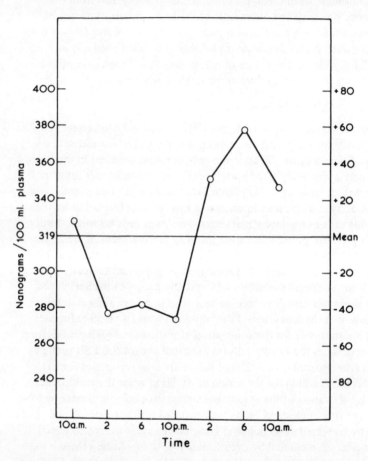

Source: Reprinted from W.P. Collins & J.F. Hennan, 'Radioimmunoassay and Reproductive Endocrinology', in H. Baum & J. Gergely (eds.), *Molecular Aspects of Medicine* (1976), vol. 1, pp. 3-128, by permission of the authors and Pergamon Press, Oxford-New York-Braunschweig.

levels do undergo a nyctohemeral rhythm (Figure 6.5), the episodic variation in testosterone secretion may well obscure this in individual subjects.

Control of Ovarian Function

The details of the development of follicles and their subsequent rupture at ovulation are well-known and will not be described here in any detail. In the human female, one follicle ripens at a time, follicular fluid accumulating between the granulosa cells; the mature follicle is known as the Graafian follicle. Rupture then occurs on the surface of the ovary and the ova pass down the Fallopian tubes, where they may be fertilised by spermatozoa from the male. The fertilised ova then become implanted in the uterine wall and divide to produce the blastocysts. Should no fertilisation occur, however, the ova pass out of the uterus.

Following ovulation the follicle collapses and is transformed into the corpus luteum, as a result of the granulosa cells proliferating and becoming vascularised. In the human female the cycle takes approximately 28 days and continues from puberty to the menopause. During the past few years, using radioimmunoassay techniques, it has been possible to measure plasma gonadotrophin and steroid-hormone levels during the menstrual cycle. By this means, a great deal has now been discovered about its hormonal control through a complex interaction between hypothalamus, anterior pituitary and ovaries (Figure 6.4). One of these (the 'long-loop feedback') occurs through raised concentrations of oestrogens and progestagens in peripheral plasma inhibiting the secretion of LH-RH/FSH-RH from the hypothalamus or from extra-hypothalamic areas of the brain. The other (the 'short-loop feedback') may occur as a result of plasma levels of LH and FSH controlling the release of LH-RH/FSH-RH.

Plasma Gonadotrophins and Steroid Hormones during the Menstrual Cycle

Figure 6.6 shows the changes in LH, FSH, oestradiol-17β, progesterone and 17α-hydroxyprogesterone during a typical menstrual cycle; adopting the common practice, the next cycle is considered to begin when menstruation starts. It is now thought that both FSH and LH, acting together with another hormone, probably prolactin, are responsible for the development and maturation of a follicle. Figure 6.6 shows that plasma levels of FSH increase to a peak early in the follicular phase, then decline and reach another peak at a much higher level at day 14. Levels of LH are relatively constant initially, but reach a maximum (the 'LH surge') at day 14. During the luteal phase, the levels of both hormones fall to the same, or slightly lower, values than in the early proliferative phase. The developing follicle synthesises and secretes oestrogens and this is born out (Figure 6.6) by the increasing plasma levels of oestradiol-17β, which peak just before the FSH/LH

Figure 6.6: Concentration of Hormones in Blood during the Menstrual Cycle

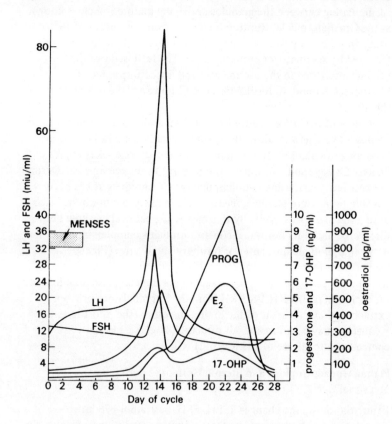

Source: Reprinted from L. Speroff & R.L. Vande Wiele, *American Journal of Obstetrics and Gynaecology* (1971), vol. 109, p. 234, by permission of the authors and the C.V. Mosby Company.

peak, on day 14. This timing is so regular that it is common practice to call this day zero and to relate all other days as − or + days. The LH surge precedes ovulation by one or two days and the peak of oestradiol-17β which occurs just prior to this is thought to mediate the mechanism for release of the mature follicle. LH is certainly necessary and the hypothalamus must be stimulated at precisely the correct time to secrete FSH-RH/LH-RH in order to stimulate LH release from the anterior pituitary. In this respect it is noteworthy that, in some cases

of infertility, ovulation can be induced by accurately timed administration of a mixture of FSH and LH over a few days, in divided doses.

As indicated earlier, after ovulation the ruptured follicle is transformed into the corpus luteum. It is possible that LH in small amounts
is responsible for the maintenance of this for about nine days; thereafter it degenerates. LH stimulates the synthesis of progesterone,
17α-hydroxyprogesterone and oestrogens by the corpus luteum and,
in many experiments, as much as 70 per cent of pregnenolone was
converted to progesterone as a result of the greatly increased activity
of the 5-ene-3β-hydroxysteroid dehydrogenase in post-ovulation
ovaries. It has also been shown that the activity of the C-17,20 lyase
activity is diminished and this is reflected (a) in rather small yields of
4-androstenedione from 17α-hydroxyprogesterone and (b) in higher
amounts of the latter, which are formed from progesterone. Figure
6.6 illustrates the massive rise in plasma progesterone and the much
smaller rise in 17α-hydroxyprogesterone. The values of oestrogen
during the luteal phase are only about one-third of those in the
follicular phase and this can be explained by the reduced quantities of
4-androstenedione/testosterone available as substrates.

Changes in the Uterine Endometrium

These are shown in Figure 6.7 in relation to the levels of plasma
steroids. During the follicular phase, oestrogens produced by the
mature follicle cause marked changes in the endometrial wall. Notably,
the wall becomes thicker, the epithelial cells become columnar and,
during the late follicular phase, the stromal layer becomes more
vascular, with the development of uterine glands. After ovulation,
the combined effects of oestrogen and progesterone from the corpus
luteum cause the stroma to become highly vascularised and the endometrial glands begin to secrete fluid into the uterus. When the corpus
luteum regresses and plasma levels of oestrogen and progesterone are
rapidly reduced, however, more intensive spiralling of the endometrial
arteries occurs, which had already begun in the follicular phase; the
arteries within the basal layer thus become constricted, causing venous
stasis and ischaemia, and bleeding commences.

Urinary Steroid Excretion throughout the Menstrual Cycle

It will be appreciated, therefore, that values for plasma progesterone,
17α-hydroxyprogesterone, oestrogens and gonadotrophins are of little
use without reference to the day of the cycle on which the blood
sample was taken. Thus, Table 6.1 indicates whether the values relate

Figure 6.7: Correlation of Changes in Plasma Concentrations of Gonadotrophins and Steroid Hormones with Changes in Ovarian and Endometrial Structure during the Menstrual Cycle

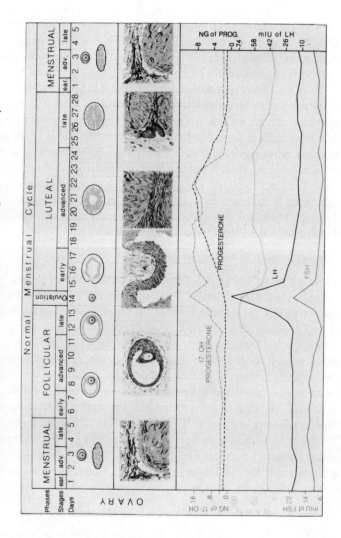

Figure 6.7—cont.

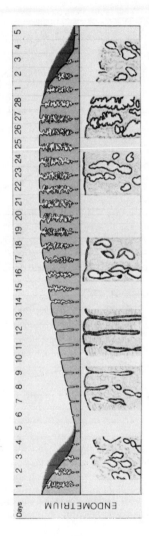

Source: Reprinted (with modification) from G.T. Ross & R.L. Vande Wiele, 'The Ovary', in R.H. Williams (ed.), *Textbook of Endocrinology*, 5th edn. (1974), pp. 368-422, by permission of the authors and W.B. Saunders & Co. Ltd., London-Philadelphia-Toronto.

Figure 6.8: Changes in the Urinary Excretion of Oestrogens, Pregnanediol and Pregnanetriol during the Menstrual Cycle

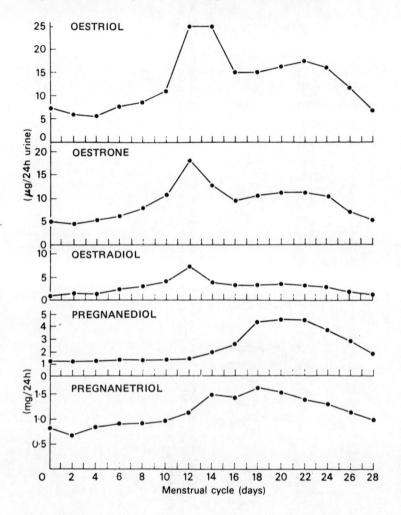

Source: Reprinted from K. Fotherby, 'The Endocrinology of the Menstrual Cycle and Pregnancy', in H.L.J. Makin (ed.), *Biochemistry of Steroid Hormones* (1975), pp. 249-72, by permission of the author and Blackwell Scientific Publications, Oxford-London-Edinburgh-Melbourne.

to the follicular or luteal phase. It is also important to do the same for urinary steroid levels. The processes whereby progesterone, 17α-hydroxyprogesterone and oestrogens are catabolised and the conjugated products excreted have been described earlier in Chapter 5. Oestrogens are excreted as their conjugates, while progesterone and 17α-hydroxyprogesterone are reduced to 5β-pregnane-3α,20α-diol (pregnanediol) and 5β-pregnane-3α,17α,20α-triol (pregnanetriol) respectively, and excreted as glucuronides. Figure 6.8 summarises the urinary excretion of these during a typical menstrual cycle. In the follicular phase, total urinary oestrogens occur at a concentration of 20-150 nmol/24 h, but the amount increases markedly during the luteal phase (45-290 nmol/24 h).

Similarly, the amounts of pregnanediol and pregnanetriol excreted during the follicular phase are low; the progesterone and 17α-hydroxyprogesterone accounting for these metabolites are generally accepted as being derived from the adrenal cortex at this time. During the luteal phase, however, the pregnanediol excretion increases almost tenfold and there is a correspondingly smaller increase in pregnanetriol excretion.

References

Collins, W.P., & Hennan, J.F., 'Radioimmunoassay and Reproductive Endocrinology', *Molecular Aspects of Medicine* (1976), vol. 1, pp. 3-128.
Fotherby, K., 'The Endocrinology of the Menstrual Cycle and Pregnancy', in H.L.J. Makin (ed.) *Biochemistry of Steroid Hormones* (Blackwell Scientific Publications, Oxford-London-Edinburgh-Melbourne, 1975), pp. 249-72.

7 METABOLISM IN PREGNANCY

The changes occurring in plasma levels of steroids during the menstrual cycle and after ovulation have been described in Chapter 6. If fertilisation has not occurred, the corpus luteum regresses and, towards the end of the luteal phase, plasma progesterone and oestrogens decrease to very low levels. If fertilisation has occurred, however, the corpus luteum continues to secrete progesterone and oestrogens so that, by the sixth week of pregnancy, plasma levels of oestradiol-17β are higher than those at the time of the luteal peak. A similar situation occurs for plasma progesterone levels by the ninth week. The increased production of 17α-hydroxyprogesterone is a feature of the corpus luteum, and measurements of this steroid in the maternal, peripheral plasma have revealed that luteal tissue persists for 9 to 10 weeks of pregnancy; at that time, the plasma 17α-hydroxyprogesterone concentration falls to similar levels as those found in the later stages of the luteal phase.

By this time, the placenta has begun to take over the production of progesterone and oestrogens from the corpus luteum. A great number of experiments have been performed during the past fifteen years to study the biosynthetic capacity of the placenta and of the foetus. Much of the information has been obtained from cases of therapeutic abortions, mainly carried out abroad and three such experiments will be described in order to give an indication of the techniques used and the conclusions drawn.

(a) In one case, the placenta was disconnected from the foetus and was perfused *in situ* with isotopically-labelled steroids, such as [^{14}C] DHA and [^{3}H] DHA sulphate (DHAS). The placental perfusate was collected and analysis revealed that approximately 70 per cent of the total radioactivity was phenolic and more than 80 per cent of this could be accounted for by oestriol, oestradiol-17β and oestrone. Isotopically-labelled oestriol was also detected in the maternal urine. This experiment clearly indicated the extraordinary capacity of the placenta to aromatise C_{19} steroids like DHA, and the following pathway was suggested:

$$\text{DHAS} \rightleftharpoons \text{DHA} \rightarrow \text{4-androstenedione} \rightleftharpoons \text{testosterone}$$
$$\downarrow \qquad\qquad\qquad\qquad \downarrow$$
$$\text{oestrone} \rightleftharpoons \text{oestradiol-17}\beta$$

(b) The second kind of experiment has consisted of injecting labelled DHA and DHAS into a uterine artery some fifteen minutes prior to therapeutic interruption of pregnancy. No radioactivity was found in the amniotic fluid, thus indicating that the radioactive steroids reached the foetus via the transplacental passage. Subsequent analysis of the placenta showed that approximately 80 per cent of the radioactive steroids was in the free form. More than 80 per cent of the radioactive steroids from the foetal tissues was shown to be phenolic and consisted almost entirely of oestrone and oestradiol-17β conjugates. These results indicated the capacity of the foetus for conjugating steroids, in contrast to the placenta.

(c) The third type of experiment has been done with normal pregnant women. [^{3}H] DHAS was injected into an ante-cubital vein and [^{14}C] DHAS into the umbilical vein. The capacity of the foetus and placenta for converting DHAS into oestrogen, mostly oestriol, was far higher than in the maternal circulation.

These experiments and many others have revealed that the foetus and placenta function as a unit in synthesising steroid hormones and complement each other in that, if a steroid-transforming enzyme is absent in one, it is present in the other. The expression 'foeto-placental unit' has therefore come into being.

Steroid Hormone Biosynthesis by the Foeto-placental Unit

Although placental tissue is unable to synthesise cholesterol from acetate, it can use maternal cholesterol as a substrate and readily convert it into pregnenolone. Foetal tissues, however, can convert acetate into cholesterol and also synthesise DHA from acetate or directly from cholesterol by removal of the side-chain. The DHA and pregnenolone so formed are rapidly sulphated by the active sulpho-kinases of the foetal adrenals, as shown by the earlier experiments (b, above). The further metabolism of these compounds in foetal and placental compartments is very complex, particularly in the formation of different steroid conjugates and of the transfer from one compartment to the other. The present account is, therefore, a simplified one.

In general terms the placenta is characterised by marked ability to convert pregnenolone to progesterone (5-ene-3β-OHSDH/isomerase system), to aromatise C_{19} compounds to oestrogens and to hydrolyse steroid sulphates (as a result of sulphatase activity). In contrast, the activities of 16α- and 17α-hydroxylases and of the C-17,20 lyase are low. Thus, in placental tissue, pregnenolone is rapidly converted to

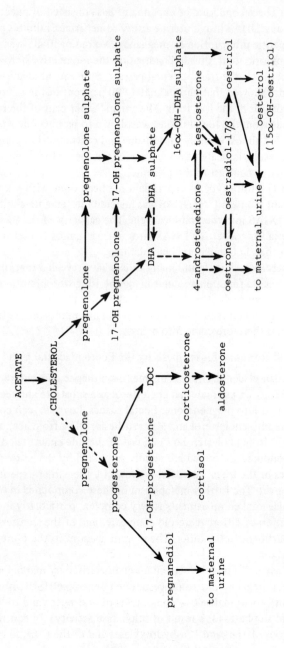

Figure 7.1: Steroid Biosynthetic Pathways (abbreviated) Occurring in the Foeto-placental Unit. Transformations occurring mainly in foetal tissues are indicated by ——→, those occurring mainly in the placenta by – – –→

progesterone but this is not metabolised further by 17α-hydroxylation and side-chain cleavage but is passed to the foetus or to the maternal tissues for further metabolism (Figure 7.1).

Unlike the placenta, foetal adrenals are characterised by their marked ability for sulphate formation, 17α-hydroxylation and C_{19} steroid side-chain cleavage (C-17,20 lyase). Pregnenolone (formed from cholesterol) is therefore rapidly converted to its sulphate, then hydroxylated to 17α-hydroxypregnenolone sulphate and thence to DHAS by side-chain cleavage. It will be recalled that cholesterol can give rise directly to DHA and this would also contribute to the foetal DHAS pool. It has been estimated that the foetal adrenals can produce as much as 100 mg of this conjugate per day. Some DHA and a considerable proportion of the DHAS are further metabolised in the foetal liver to 16α-hydroxy derivatives; this ability is a specific characteristic of foetal tissues since placenta possesses no 16α-hydroxylase.

DHA, DHAS and their 16α-hydroxy derivatives are then transferred back to the placenta where the conjugates are hydrolysed by sulphatases and the free steroids are converted by 5-ene-3β-OHSDH/isomerase to 4-androstenedione and 16α-hydroxy-4-androstenedione, respectively. Finally, aromatisation results in oestrone, oestradiol-17β and, especially, oestriol from the 16α-hydroxy derivative. Quantitatively, oestriol is the most important oestrogen synthesised in the foeto-placental unit (Figure 7.1), its concentration in urine being about 100 times that of oestradiol-17β or oestrone.

In addition to its other activities, the foetal adrenals can convert progesterone (derived from the placenta) to deoxycorticosterone and thence to corticosterone and aldosterone. The cortisol pathway occurs by way of 17α-hydroxylation of progesterone and by the pathways described in Chapter 3. As a result of the combined function of placenta and foetus, progesterone and oestrogens are synthesised in considerable amounts, especially in the second half of pregnancy. The majority of the progesterone is catabolised to pregnanediol and excreted in the maternal urine, as the glucuronide conjugate (see Chapter 5). Figures 7.2 and 7.3 summarise the changes in plasma levels of progesterone and oestrogens, and the urinary excretion of pregnanediol and oestrogens during pregnancy. It can be seen that, in some cases, as much as 70 mg per day of pregnanediol and 35 mg per day of oestriol are excreted in maternal urine just before term. These enormous quantities are some 100 and 1000 times, respectively, greater than the amounts excreted during the follicular stage of the menstrual cycle. Serial estimations of plasma or urinary oestriol during the later

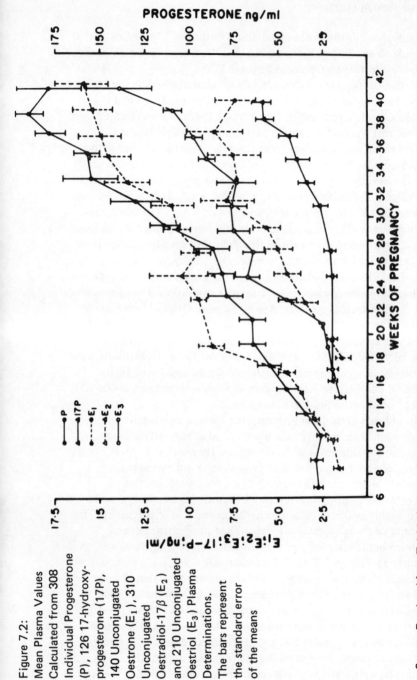

Figure 7.2:
Mean Plasma Values
Calculated from 308
Individual Progesterone
(P), 126 17-hydroxy-
progesterone (17P),
140 Unconjugated
Oestrone (E_1), 310
Unconjugated
Oestradiol-17β (E_2)
and 210 Unconjugated
Oestriol (E_3) Plasma
Determinations.
The bars represent
the standard error
of the means

Source: Reprinted from Tulchinsky et al., American Journal of Obstetrics and Gynaecology (1972), vol. 112, pp. 1095-1100, by permission of the authors and the C.V. Mosby Company.

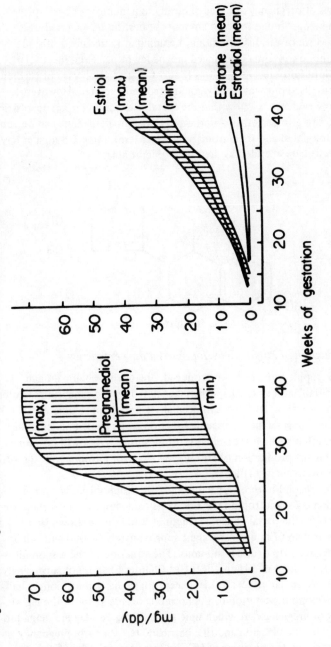

Figure 7.3: Changes in Urinary Levels of Pregnanediol and Oestrogens during Pregnancy

Source: Reprinted from D. Schulster, S. Burstein & B.A. Cooke, *Molecular Endocrinology of the Steroid Hormones* (1976), p. 153, by permission of Dr Cooke and John Wiley & Sons, London-New York-Sydney-Toronto.

stages of pregnancy are used clinically as a monitor of foeto-placental well-being. Should lowered amounts of oestriol be excreted, it is suggestive of various situations, including intra-uterine death, pre-eclamptic toxaemia, prolonged pregnancy or placental insufficiency.

Until fairly recently, it was thought that oestriol was not further metabolised but was merely conjugated and excreted. However, there is now evidence to show that the foetal liver can hydroxylate oestriol at C-15α to give oestetrol. Alternatively, 4-androstenedione can be 15α-hydroxylated and then aromatised. Near term, some 2.5 mg per day of oestetrol are excreted as the ring D glucuronide.

oestetrol

Production of Polypeptide Hormones during Pregnancy

Two trophic hormones are produced, one of these being human placental lactogen (HPL), which is secreted by the syncytiotrophoblast of the placenta. HPL has a molecular weight of approximately 21 000 and has considerable lactogenic function, as its name implies. It also has other effects which are similar to those shown by growth hormone. The rate of production of HPL increases steadily from about the fifth week of pregnancy (Figure 7.4).

The second hormone, produced by the trophoblast, is human chorionic gonadotrophin (HCG). As its name implies, it exerts powerful effects on the foetal gonads. Structural studies have shown that it is a glycoprotein of molecular weight approximately 30 000 and can be dissociated into α- and β-sub-units. The structure of the α-sub-unit is similar to those of LH and FSH (see Chapter 6) and, not surprisingly, HCG has similar effects to LH, except that it has a much longer half-life. Maximum secretion of the hormone occurs at about the eighth week of pregnancy, at which time some 26 mg per day are being produced by the placenta and the diagnostic test for early pregnancy relies on detecting the presence of HCG in the maternal urine. From the

Figure 7.4: Relationship between Serum Human Placental Lactogen (HPL), Placental Weight and Time of Gestation

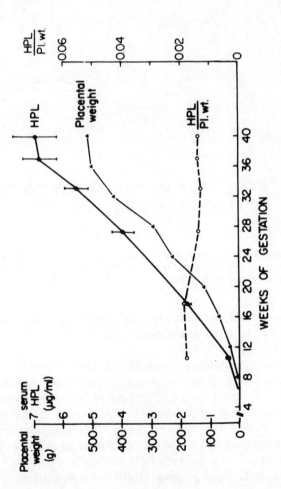

Source: Reprinted from H.A. Selenkow et al., 'Measurement and Pathophysiologic Significance of Human Placental Lactogen', in A. Pecile & C. Finzi (eds.), The Foeto-placental Unit (1969), pp. 340-62, by permission of the authors and Excerpta Medica Foundation, London-Amsterdam.

Figure 7.5: Mean Serum Level of Human Chorionic Gonadotrophin (HCG) during Pregnancy. The curves are based on results reported by various authors using different bioassay and immunoassay methods: (1) uterine weight increase in rats; (2) ovarian hyperaemia in rats; (3) complement fixation; (4) haemagglutinin inhibition

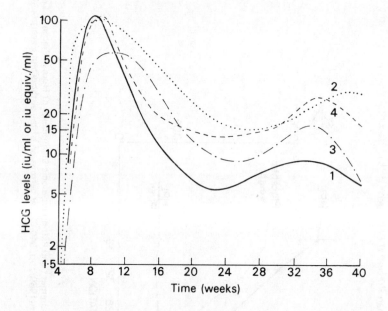

Source: Reprinted from R. Borth, 'Chorionic Gonadotrophin', in F. Fuchs & A. Klopper (eds.), *Endocrinology of Pregnancy* (1971), pp. 16-31, by permission of the author and Harper & Row, Publishers, New York-London.

eighth week onwards, the production rate decreases to a minimum by about 20 weeks, followed by a secondary, much smaller peak around weeks 32 to 33 (Figure 7.5).

With the advent of radioimmunoassay, it has been possible to measure foetal peripheral plasma testosterone levels and to study the control of gonadal function by LH, FSH and HCG. Androgen secretion by the foetal testis is thought to be under the influence of HCG and begins at about the sixth week of pregnancy. The maximum testosterone levels occur at twelve weeks, followed by a decline, reflected in the decline in placental HCG production. Following the actions of HCG, foetal pituitary LH stimulates testosterone

Figure 7.6: Pattern of Serum LH, FSH, hCG and Testosterone and of Pituitary LH and FSH in the Male Human Foetus during Gestation as Integrated with the Developmental Histology of the Foetal Testis

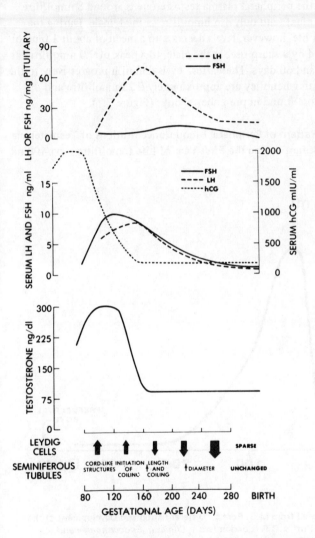

Source: Reprinted from S.L. Kaplan & M.M. Grumbach, 'Gonadotrophins and Sex Steroids in the Foetus', in G.T. Ross & M.B. Lipsett (eds.), *Clinics in Endocrinology and Metabolism* (1978), vol. 7, pp. 487-511, by permission of the authors and W.B. Saunders & Co. Ltd., London-Philadelphia-Toronto.

synthesis necessary for development of the genitalia; the development
of the tubules and Sertoli cells is under the control of the foetal
pituitary FSH (Figure 7.6).

At birth, the peripheral plasma testosterone is around 8 nmol/litre
in the male infant, and only 1.5 nmol/litre in the female. During the
first week of life, however, levels decrease to a mean of about 1.0 nmol/
litre followed by a sharp rise, in the male, to a peak of 9.0 nmol/litre at
between 30 and 60 days. Thereafter, levels diminish progressively to the
seventh month when they are approximately 0.25 nmol/litre and
similar to those found in pre-pubertal boys (Figure 7.7).

Figure 7.7: Pattern of Peripheral Blood Concentrations of Testosterone
in the Male Infant during the First Year of Life (nmol/litre = ng/100 ml
x 0.035)

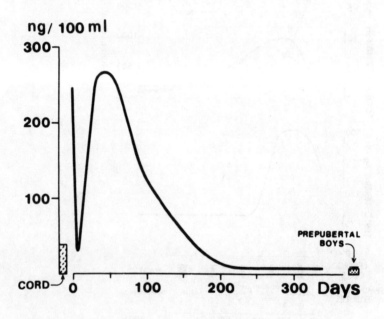

Source: Reprinted from M.G. Forest, 'Differentiation and Development of the
Male', in W.R. Butt & D.R. London (eds.), *Clinics in Endocrinology and
Metabolism* (1975), vol. 4, pp. 569-96, by permission of the author and W.B.
Saunders & Co. Ltd., London-Philadelphia-Toronto.

Contraceptive Steroids

Research into contraception has been pursued since the latter part of
the nineteenth century. Studies during the 1930s showed that injections of oestrogens and progesterone (steroids which were being newly
isolated at that time from biological sources) could inhibit ovulation
in animals. The effects of these steroids, however, were short-lived
due to their relatively rapid inactivation. Thus, a search began for
synthetic compounds which would have similar, or more powerful,
effects as the endogenous steroids but would retain their potency for
at least 24 hours.

Oestrogenic Compounds

It is generally accepted that these possess contraceptive activity by
virtue of the fact that they inhibit ovulation by interfering with the
elaboration of gonadotrophin-releasing hormones from the hypothalamus (see p. 73); the ovaries therefore become quiescent.

The first compound to be synthesised, which had oestrogenic properties, was stilboestrol. However, it was later discovered that structural
modifications of oestradiol-17β itself (Figure 7.8) prolonged the life of
the molecule. Ethynyloestradiol has a 17α-ethynyl group ($- - - C \equiv CH$)
(compare the structure of norethynodrel, Figure 7.8), while
mestranol has the same structure as ethynyloestradiol except that the
hydroxyl group at C-3 is methylated ($-OCH_3$). Both these compounds
have similar oestrogenic effects to those of oestradiol-17β but, in the
case of ethynyloestradiol, a dose of only 60 μg by mouth is active for
24-36 hours.

Progestagens

In addition to those possessing oestrogenic properties, a number of
compounds have been synthesised which have progesterone-like
properties and which are widely used as oral contraceptives. One group
(Figure 7.8) consists of compounds derived from 19-*nor*testosterone,
that is, testosterone which lacks the usual angular methyl group at
C-10. The presence of the ethynyl substituent at C-17 is a structural
feature that is common to all the members of this group, and it is this,
together with the lack of the angular methyl group, which makes these
compounds more potent ovulation suppressors than those derived
from 17α-hydroxyprogesterone. Figure 7.8 also illustrates the
structures of this group of progestagens. It is particularly interesting
that 17α-hydroxyprogesterone itself has no contraceptive action when
administered orally but esterification of the 17-hydroxyl group results

Figure 7.8: Structural Formulae of (upper) 19-Nortestosterone Derivatives and (lower) 17α-Hydroxyprogesterone Derivatives Used in Steroidal Contraception

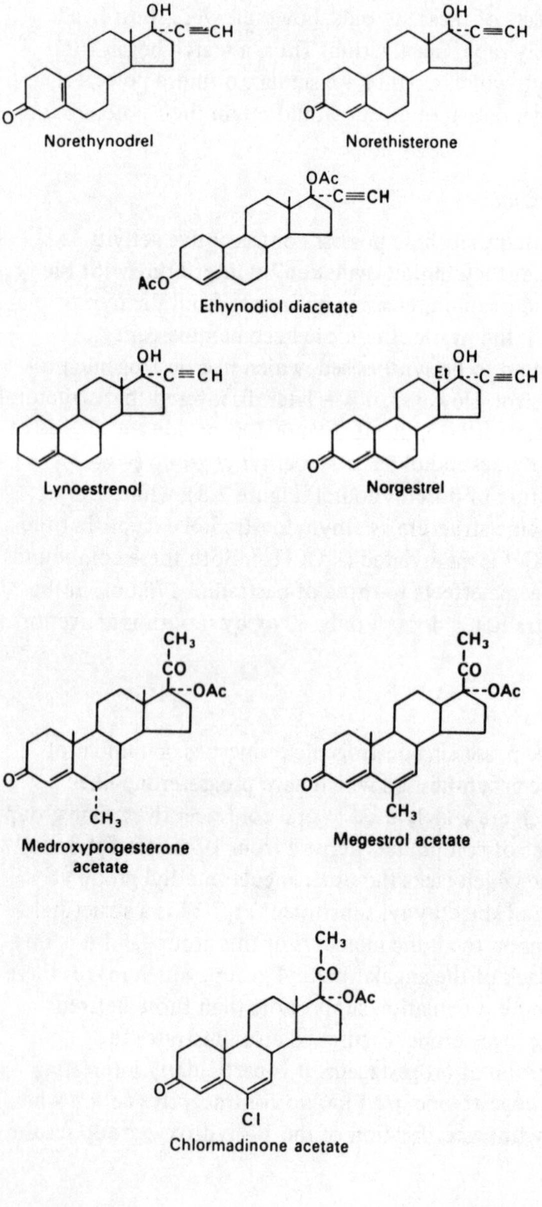
OH
C≡CH
Norethynodrel
OH
C≡CH
Norethisterone
OAc
C≡CH
AcO
Ethynodiol diacetate
OH
C≡CH
Lynoestrenol
OH
Et
C≡CH
Norgestrel
CH₃
CO
OAc
CH₃
Medroxyprogesterone acetate
CH₃
CO
OAc
CH₃
Megestrol acetate
CH₃
CO
OAc
Cl
Chlormadinone acetate

in a compound that has similar actions to progesterone; further substitutions in the molecule enhance progestational activity. Such progestagens induce the formation of scanty, viscoid cervical mucus so that sperm motility and penetration are hindered. They are also able to maintain the endometrium, thus preventing its breakdown and the accompanying bleeding. In addition, progestagens act synergistically with oestrogens on the hypothalamus. For a more extensive review of this subject, the reader is referred to Kleinman (1973).

Reference

Kleinman, R.L. (ed.), *Systemic Contraception* (International Planned Parenthood Federation, London, 1973).

8 DISORDERS OF STEROIDOGENESIS

The pathways of biosynthesis of steroid hormones and their control mechanisms have been described in earlier chapters. There are a number of pathological conditions, however, which lead to changes in pituitary-adrenal function. In addition, some inborn errors of adrenal steroid production are well-documented. These situations will be explained briefly here under the headings of adrenocortical hypo- and hyper-function. For a fuller description, the reader is referred to the accounts by Besser & Edwards (1972), Hamilton (1972), James (1975) and Edwards (1975) and to the book by Schulster, Burstein & Cooke (1976).

Adrenocortical Hypofunction

Two conditions are recognised in which the ability of the adrenal cortex to synthesise steroid hormones is deficient.

(a) Primary Adrenal Insufficiency

This is known as Addison's disease and occurs through partial or complete destruction of all three zones of the cortex, usually as a result of autoimmune disease. The production of all adrenal steroid hormones is decreased, with plasma steroid levels and urinary excretion of reduced steroid metabolites all diminished, sometimes to only 20 per cent of the normal values. As a result of the lowered plasma cortisol levels, the normal 'feedback' inhibition of hypothalamic CRF secretion is reduced, thus allowing the anterior pituitary to produce excessive quantities of ACTH, which maximally stimulate the adrenals. In some cases, grossly excessive plasma levels of ACTH have been recorded. This can be shown clearly in Addisonian patients by injecting ACTH; no change occurs in plasma cortisol levels whereas, in normal patients, the adrenals respond by increased synthesis of cortisol (see Chapter 6). There are various other clinical symptoms in Addison's disease associated with the lack of cortisol and aldosterone, such as hypoglycaemia and lowered plasma sodium ion and chloride ion, with hypotension. In addition, the high plasma levels of melanocyte-stimulating hormone (MSH), which is secreted along with ACTH, may lead to skin pigmentation. Treatment consists of administration of both glucocorticoids, such as prednisolone, and mineralocorticoids, such as 9α-fluorocortisol.

(b)   Secondary Adrenal Insufficiency

In this condition, the lesion is sometimes at the level of the hypothalamus or, more usually, lies with the anterior pituitary, which does not therefore secrete ACTH to stimulate the otherwise normal adrenals. As a result, the production of glucocorticosteroids is diminished but the secretion of aldosterone is unaffected, because ACTH has only minor stimulatory effects on this pathway. As would be expected, plasma ACTH levels are very low (less than 1 mU/ml or 10 pg/ml) and, in contrast to primary adrenal insufficiency, an injection of ACTH increases plasma and urinary steroid levels.

Adrenocortical Hyperfunction

Cushing's disease (named after the investigator who first described it) results from excessive cortisol production by the adrenals. Such a situation can occur in any one of three ways. First, hyperplasia of adrenocortical tissue and overproduction of steroids can result from an ACTH-secreting adenoma of the anterior pituitary. Secondly, an autonomous adrenal tumour can produce excessive quantities of steroids, thereby reducing the secretion of ACTH from the pituitary. This results in understimulation of the normal, contra-lateral adrenal, which atrophies. If the tumour is benign (adenoma), cortisol is the major steroid formed but, if a malignant tumour (carcinoma) is present, then a range of steroid hormones is produced, often in massive quantities. Thirdly, the site of ACTH production may be an ACTH-secreting tumour in non-endocrine tissues, commonly in the lung. This condition is known as the 'ectopic ACTH syndrome'.

The effects of cortisol have already been described in Chapter 2 and, in Cushing's disease, diminished protein synthesis means that some areas of skin (known as striae) are thin, with blood vessels showing through. The vessel walls become fragile so that bruising is a common feature. Muscular weakness is also apparent. As expected also, disorders of carbohydrate metabolism occur with the patient showing the symptoms of diabetes with impaired glucose tolerance and glycosuria. Abnormalities of lipid metabolism are manifested in the characteristic fat, red 'moonface' and a protuberant abdomen. Hirsutism is sometimes present, particularly so in women with an adrenocortical carcinoma, as a result of the overproduction of adrenal androgens.

Figure 8.1: Circadian Rhythm of Plasma Fluorogenic Corticosteroids in One Normal Subject, Two Patients with Cushing's Disease and One Patient with an Adrenal Adenoma and Cushing's Syndrome

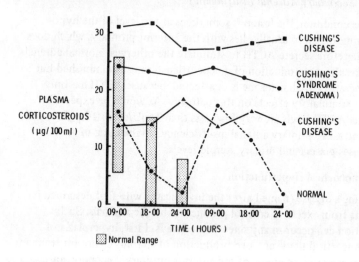

Source: Reprinted from G.M. Besser & C.R.W. Edwards, 'Cushing's Syndrome', in A.S. Mason (ed.), *Clinics in Endocrinology and Metabolism* (1972), vol. 1, pp. 451-501, by permission of the authors and W.B. Saunders & Co. Ltd., London-Philadelphia-Toronto.

In these situations, plasma cortisol levels are usually high and the normal nyctohemeral rhythm is lost (Figure 8.1); as would be expected, the excretion of 17-oxogenic steroids is also raised. If ACTH is administered acutely, there is little or no increase in plasma cortisol levels, in keeping with the fact that the feedback mechanism no longer operates and that the situation is outside the normal endocrine control. In a similar way, in patients with adrenocortical tumour or the ectopic ACTH syndrome, there is virtually no suppression of adrenal function in response to dexamethasone; in normal subjects, however, this inhibits ACTH release and results in a marked diminution of plasma cortisol levels. In patients with Cushing's disease, the dexamethasone suppression test (as it is called) is only partially effective.

Abnormalities of Aldosterone Biosynthesis

Reduced production of aldosterone can occur in Addison's disease because of damage to the cells of the zona glomerulosa, and also in congenital adrenal hyperplasia where there is a deficiency of relevant enzymes (see below).

Hyperaldosteronism can occur as a result of aldosterone-producing adenomas in a syndrome known as Conn's syndrome, after the investigator who first described the condition. The increased aldosterone levels in the plasma will inhibit renin release, by the feedback mechanisms described in Chapter 6, and both plasma renin and angiotensin levels will be lowered. The overall results of the condition are that sodium ion is retained, potassium ion is lost in the urine and there is hypertension. The accepted treatment for such patients is surgical removal of the adenoma and for those for whom surgery is undesirable, spironolactone is given to block the actions of aldosterone on the distal renal tubules.

Inborn Errors of Corticosteroid Biosynthesis

A number of enzymes involved in corticosteroid biosynthesis (see Chapter 3) are now known to be deficient in a small number of individuals through genetic errors, which are inherited as autosomal (non sex-linked) characteristics; thus, both sexes are affected equally. A deficiency in one or more enzymes for cortisol synthesis will, of course, result in excessive production of ACTH and further stimulation of the inefficient adrenals. They therefore become hyperplastic and the disorders have come to be known collectively as 'congenital adrenal hyperplasia' (CAH). With respect to live births, the incidence of CAH in differing populations varies from 1 in 5000 to 1 in 67 000.

The 21-Hydroxylase Defect

This is the most common defect, accounting for 95 per cent of all cases of CAH reported. Figure 8.2 shows that progesterone is not 21-hydroxylated to deoxycorticosterone (DOC) nor is 17α-hydroxyprogesterone converted to 11-deoxycortisol. As indicated above, the lowered plasma cortisol levels will result in excessive stimulation of the adrenals by ACTH. Furthermore, progesterone and 17α-hydroxyprogesterone accumulate, and are metabolised via the alternative route available to them to give rise to androgens. The possible overproduction of C_{19} steroids, such as 4-androstenedione and testosterone, can cause virilism. Since the major catabolite of 17α-hydroxyprogesterone is pregnanetriol (see Chapter 5), the urinary excretion of this, as well as of the 17-oxosteroids (derived from the androgens), is greatly increased.

Two variants of the 21-hydroxylase defect are recognised — the 'non salt-losing' and 'salt-losing' types. The former probably arises

Figure 8.2: Enzymic Blocks in Congenital Adrenal Hyperplasia. ⑪ indicates the position of hydroxylation; OHSDH means hydroxysteroid dehydrogenase

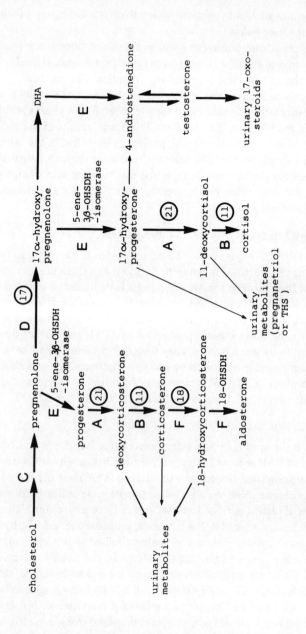

because only the 21-hydroxylase which resides in the cells of the zona reticularis and zona fasciculata is affected, whereas in the 'salt-losing' type the 21-hydroxylase of the zona glomerulosa is also affected and results in impairment of aldosterone biosynthesis.

The 11β-Hydroxylase Defect

The second most common defect is that involving 11β-hydroxylase, although only about 4 per cent of all CAH cases are thus characterised. In this situation, 11-deoxycortisol and deoxycorticosterone cannot be converted to cortisol and corticosterone, respectively, by 11β-hydroxylation (Figure 8.2). Once again the anterior pituitary is allowed to secrete excessive quantities of ACTH because of the diminished cortisol production. The catabolite of 11-deoxycortisol (substance S), formed by the reductive processes described earlier (Chapter 5), is $3\alpha,17\alpha,21$-trihydroxy-5β-pregnan-20-one (THS) and the presence of this in urine, together with the finding of a raised plasma 11-deoxycortisol relative to cortisol, are good indications that the defect lies in the 11β-hydroxylase. The hypertension found in these patients may be due to high plasma levels of DOC, because this steroid has pronounced mineralocorticoid properties. Virilism is another feature of the disorder and this undoubtedly arises from excessive adrenal androgen production from 17α-hydroxypregnenolone and 17α-hydroxyprogesterone. Both the 21- and 11β-hydroxylase defects can be treated with glucocorticoids.

The remainder of the enzyme defects in CAH together account for only 1 per cent of the recorded cases. The following enzymes can be affected:

(1) an enzyme, or enzymes, between colesterol and pregnenolone, when the adrenals are greatly enlarged and the cells are laden with cholesterol;

(2) 17α-hydroxylase, in which case the adrenals are unable to synthesise 17-hydroxylated corticosteroids, such as cortisol, but instead are stimulated by ACTH to produce 17-deoxysteroids, such as deoxycorticosterone, corticosterone and aldosterone. Androgen biosynthesis is also deficient because 17α-hydroxylation of pregnenolone and progesterone is an essential requirement before side-chain cleavage can occur to DHA and 4-androstenedione;

(3) 18-hydroxylase and 18-hydroxysteroid dehydrogenase, in which case affected individuals exhibit a deficiency in aldosterone biosynthesis and salt loss; the production of glucocorticoids and of androgens appears normal;

(4) 5-ene-3β-hydroxysteroid dehydrogenase/isomerase. In these patients pregnenolone is prevented from being converted to progesterone, so that the 5-ene-3β-hydroxysteroid pathway is taken preferentially, leading to the formation of 17α-hydroxypregnenolone, DHA and 5-androstenediol. The urine contains steroid catabolites of the 5-en-3β-hydroxy configuration, such as 5-pregnenediol, and the 17-oxosteroid fraction contains, predominantly, DHAS. As expected, characteristic features of the condition are reduced cortisol and aldosterone synthesis (both 4-en-3-oxosteroids), resulting in salt loss. The defect, which appears to lie in the dehydrogenase rather than in the associated isomerase, manifests itself within the first few days of life and is invariably fatal.

Virilisation in Utero. The production of foetal androgens and their effects have been described in Chapter 7. In the absence of androgens, female (Müllerian) development occurs *in utero*, whereas male (Wolffian) development takes place if they are present. If the foetal adrenals have enzyme defects, such as those described above, then the cortisol precursors which accumulate in varying quantities can be converted to 11-deoxygenated androgens by side-chain cleavage; it will be remembered from what was said in Chapter 5 that this mode of catabolism accounts for some 10 per cent of corticosteroids. This means, therefore, that a female child can be born with varying degrees of virilisation, commonly with clitoral hypertrophy, often with labio-scrotal fusion. It should be remembered also that, although CAH is usually thought of as affecting infants and small children, the disease can result in problems in later life. Sometimes, females have been raised as boys or, alternatively, the occurrence of hirsutism and dysmenorrhea in women may be attributable to adrenal enzyme defects. In the male, excess androgen production *in utero* may be manifested later by precocious sexual development.

References

Besser, G.M. & Edwards, C.R.W., 'Cushing's Syndrome', in D.S.B. Inglis (ed.), *Clinics in Endocrinology and Metabolism* (W.B. Saunders & Co. Ltd., Eastbourne,-Philadelphia-Toronto, 1972), pp. 451-501.
Edwards, R.W.H., 'Inborn Errors of Corticosteroids', in H.L.J. Makin (ed.), *Biochemistry of Steroid Hormones* (Blackwell Scientific Publications, Oxford-London-Edinburgh-Melbourne, 1975), pp. 273-87.

Hamilton, W., 'Congenital Adrenal Hyperplasia', in D.S.B. Inglis (ed.), *Clinics in Endocrinology and Metabolism* (W.B. Saunders & Co. Ltd., Eastbourne-Philadelphia-Toronto, 1972), pp. 503-47.

James, V.H.T., 'Physiology and Pathology of the Pituitary-adrenal Axis', in H.L.J. Makin (ed.), *Biochemistry of Steroid Hormones* (Blackwell Scientific Publications, Oxford-London-Edinburgh-Melbourne, 1975), pp. 227-47.

Schulster, D., Burstein, S. & Cooke, B.A., *Molecular Endocrinology of the Steroid Hormones* (John Wiley & Sons, London-New York-Sydney-Toronto, 1976), pp. 98-115.

INDEX

Numbers in *italics* refer to Figures or Tables